One Word From God
Can Change
Your Health

One Word From God
Can Change
Your Health

By Kenneth and Gloria Copeland

Harrison House
Tulsa, Oklahoma

One Word From God Can Change Your Health

30-0710

07 06 05 04 03 02 01 00 99 98   10 9 8 7 6 5 4 3 2 1

One Word From God Can Change Your Health
ISBN 1-57794-145-4
Copyright © 1999 by Kenneth and Gloria Copeland
Kenneth Copeland Ministries
Fort Worth, Texas 76192-0001

Published by Harrison House, Inc.
P.O. Box 35035
Tulsa, Oklahoma 74153

Contents

Introduction

One Word From God Can Change Your Life FOREVER!

When the revelation of this statement exploded on the inside of me, it changed the way I think...about everything! I had been praying for several days about a situation that seemed at the time to be overwhelming. I had been confessing the Word of God over it, but that Word had begun to come out of my head and not my heart. I was pushing in my flesh for the circumstance to change. As I made my confession one more time, the Spirit of God seemed to say to me, *Why don't you be quiet?!*

I said, "But Lord, I'm confessing the Word!"

He answered inside me, *I know it. I heard you. Now just be still and be quiet a little while, and let the Word of God settle down in your spirit. Quit trying to make this thing happen. You're not God.*

You're not going to be the one to make it happen anyway!

So I stopped. I stopped in that situation in my mind and began to get quiet before the Lord...and this phrase came up in my spirit..."**One word from God can change anything.**"

So I started saying that. I said it off and on all day. It came easily because it came from God—not from my own thinking.

Every time I was tempted to worry or think of ideas concerning my circumstances, I'd think, *Yes, just one word from God...*

I noticed when I'd say that, **the peace of God** would come on me. It was so calming. As a result, a habit developed in me. People would bring me issues. They'd say, "Well, what about...." And I'd either say aloud or think to myself, "**Yeah, that may be so, but one word from God will change anything.**"

It began to be the answer for everything. If I was watching television and the newscaster was telling about a disaster, and the people being interviewed were saying things to the effect of "Oh, what are we going to do? It's all been blown away, burned up or shook up...," I'd say, **"Yeah, but one word from God can change anything."**

It really developed into a strength for me and it can for you. That's why we've put together the **One Word From God Book Series**...there could be just one word in these inspiring articles that can change your health forever.

You've been searching, seeking help... and God has the answer. He has the one word that can turn your circumstance around and put you on dry ground. He has the one word that gives you all the peace that's in Him. He is your Healer. He wants you to have a strong, healthy body. He wants you to live and not die, and declare the works of the Lord. (Psalm 118:17)

God loves you. And He has a word for you. One Word that can change your life FOREVER!

Kenneth Copeland

The Great Exchange

"Surely he hath borne our griefs, and carried our sorrows: yet we did esteem him stricken, smitten of God, and afflicted."
— ISAIAH 53:4

Kenneth
Copeland

Your days of sickness and disease are over.

I'll never forget the day God spoke those words to me. It was some of the best news I'd ever heard. I believed it and have been walking in the glorious truth of it for more than 25 years now.

If you're sitting there right now, wishing God would say those same words to you, I have good news for you: He has.

He has said it to every one of us.

He said it with such power and force that it made hell tremble and heaven ring. He wrote it in the covenant blood of His own Son. He shouted it down through the ages through prophets and apostles and preachers.

The problem is, most Christians haven't truly heard it. They haven't let it reach down into their hearts and become truth to them. God has said it...but they haven't yet believed.

If that is the case with you today, I want you to know that what you are about to read can change that forever. If you will take this message, study it out in the Scriptures and see for yourself that it is the truth, if you will dare to believe it and act on it, it will not only change your heart, it will change your body.

This one message will forever alter how you see sickness and disease. It will put to rest every doubt about God's will for your healing and open the door of divine health to you.

A Supernatural Substitution

What message could possibly be that powerful?

Only one. The message of the Cross.

If you're a believer, you've already experienced how life-changing that message can be. When you first received it by faith, the anointing of God in it snatched you out of the kingdom of darkness and delivered you into the kingdom of the light of God's Son. It changed your eternal destination from hell to heaven. It transformed you spiritually and made you a new creation. Think of the power it released in your life!

Yet the fact is, most of us have understood only a tiny fraction of what was accomplished at Calvary. We have only begun to grasp all that was done for us in that Great Exchange.

I like the phrase, The Great Exchange, because the Spirit of the Lord gave it to me, and it captures what happened during Jesus' death and resurrection. It communicates that Jesus did more than pour out His life to pay the penalty of our sin. He actually was made *"to be sin for us, who knew no sin; that we might be made the righteousness of God in him"* (2 Corinthians 5:21).

To understand how all-encompassing The Great Exchange truly was, you have to realize that the word *sin* there does not just refer to what we'd normally think of as religious errors. It includes everything in our lives that falls short of the glory and perfection of God's original design (see Romans 3:23).

If you want to see that original design, look back at the Garden of Eden. What you'll find is a man and a woman living in unbroken fellowship with Almighty God, untouched by sickness, grief or poverty, and exercising dominion over the whole earth.

Religion has tried to cheapen what Jesus did for us by teaching that He only brought forth a partial redemption—that He freed us only from the eternal damnation caused by sin and not from its damnable effects in the here and now. But thank God, that is not the case.

Calvary was the most complete event that has ever taken place.

God left nothing out of it. Not one cursed thing that came about through mankind's union with Satan was left standing. Jesus triumphed over it all. By taking upon Himself every foul thing that fallen man has ever suffered, He set us free—spirit, soul and body.

He became our substitute. He became poor, that we might be rich (2 Corinthians 8:9).

He became weak so that we might be strong. He endured death so that we might be made alive (1 Corinthians 15:22). He *"[bore] our sins in his own body on the tree, that we, being dead to sins, should live unto right-eousness: by whose stripes [we] were healed"* (1 Peter 2:24).

A Mystery Hidden in God

Notice there that Peter lists redemption from sin and healing in the same breath. So does Psalm 103. It says, *"Bless the Lord, O my soul: and all that is within me, bless his holy name. Bless the Lord, O my soul, and forget not all his benefits: Who forgiveth all thine iniquities; who healeth all thy diseases"* (verses 1-3).

All through the Bible, healing and forgive-ness go together like hand and glove. God does not separate them. The reason is simple. They are not separate!

Just as sickness entered the world through Adam's sin, healing came when Jesus paid the price for that sin. To believe otherwise would be tantamount to saying that what

God did in Jesus on the cross was less powerful than what the devil did in Adam in the Garden of Eden. That could not possibly be so! For Romans 5:15 assures us:

> ...God's free gift is not at all to be compared to the trespass—His grace is out of all proportion to the fall of man. For if many died through one man's falling away—his lapse, his offense—much more profusely did God's grace and the free gift [that comes] through the undeserved favor of the one Man Jesus Christ [the Anointed One], abound and overflow to and for [the benefit of] many (*The Amplified Bible*).

In other words, what God accomplished through redemption not only equaled what Satan accomplished through the Fall...it far surpassed it!

I'll admit, judging by the sickness-ridden, poverty-plagued, defeated lives of many Christians, it may not seem like redemption did much more than save us from hell by the skin of our teeth. But that's because for the most part, we don't have any idea what really happened at Calvary. And that lack of knowledge has destroyed many precious Christian lives.

"Well now, Brother Copeland, I know what happened at Calvary. I've read every Gospel account of it."

That may be so, but quite frankly, you can't find out what happened there strictly by reading Matthew, Mark, Luke and John. For one thing, those books contain very little information about the Crucifixion. And for another thing, the men who wrote them had viewed it from a natural perspective. They didn't understand it themselves at the time it happened because it was a mystery hidden in God (see 1 Corinthians 2:6-8).

To see the Crucifixion from God's perspective, you must read what the prophet Isaiah wrote about it. For God revealed to him not just the physical facts, but also the spiritual truths of what actually occurred the day Jesus died for us. You can find what he wrote in Isaiah 53:

Surely He has borne our griefs— sickness, weakness and distress—

and carried our sorrows and pain [of punishment]. Yet we ignorantly considered Him stricken, smitten and afflicted by God [as if with leprosy]. But He was wounded for our transgressions, He was bruised for our guilt and iniquities; the chastisement needful to obtain peace and well-being for us was upon Him, and with the stripes that wounded Him we are healed and made whole (verses 4-5, *The Amplified Bible*).

Some theologians have tried to rob this passage of its full power by teaching that the healing it refers to is merely spiritual healing. But the Gospel writer Matthew makes it clear that they are mistaken. For in Matthew 8:17, he quotes this very passage and applies it to the healing ministry of Jesus in which people were cured of every kind of physical sickness and disease.

With that said, look back at those scriptures again. Do you see there where it says He *"was bruised for our guilt and iniquities...and with the stripes that wounded Him we are healed"*? If you were to look up the Hebrew words that have been translated *bruised* and *stripes*, you'd find out that they both come from the same word saying He was bruised for our iniquities and with those bruises we are healed.

That means healing and forgiveness of sin were bought by the same blood that poured from the same wounds on Jesus' body. He paid the same awesome price for them both. He took on His own body every sickness and infirmity of every man just as He took on Himself the sin of every man. He suffered the torments of them all so that we could be free of them all.

The very thought of it staggers the mind. Just imagine, for a moment, if someone were to take every illness ever experienced by anyone in your city—everything from hangnails to the measles to cancer— and put them on one person all at once. It's hard to even think of such a thing, isn't it? We've never seen anybody that sick!

Imagine that same person must also take into his spirit every sin ever committed by anyone in your city. Violence, adultery, perversion, murder, hatred, jealousy, resentment—all of it must enter into him at once. Can you imagine what that would do to someone? Sin is powerful! It will change the color of a person's hair. It will twist their countenance. It will darken the light in their eyes.

Now expand that picture to include the sicknesses and sins of every man, woman and child who will ever live on this planet. Of course, you cannot imagine such horror. But if you could, you would be able to see the awful price Jesus paid for us at Calvary.

Isaiah described the sight of it, saying, *"[the Servant of God became an object of horror; many were astonished.] His face and His whole appearance were marred more than any man's, and His form beyond that of the sons of men"* (Isaiah 52:14, The Amplified Bible).

The weight of all that sin and sickness on one man was so heavy it rocked the earth. It was so terrible the sun refused to shine on it. No wonder the Roman centurion who witnessed Jesus' crucifixion said, *"Truly this man was the Son of God"* (Mark 15:39). He had never seen a man die like that.

"If It Be Thy Will"

In the light of such a sacrifice, it is as grievous to the heart of God for us to pray, "If it be Thy will, heal me," as it is for us to say, "If it be Thy will, save me." God revealed His will once and for all when He laid our sicknesses on Jesus. Giving us that revelation cost Him dearly. Once, when He spoke to me of Calvary, He said, *It is as close to Me as if it had happened today. It is burned into My consciousness.*

How dare we, then, ignore what happened there and tell some sick brother that it is God's will for him to be sick a little longer so he can learn something?

Isaiah 53:10 says, *"It was the will of the Lord to bruise Him; He has put Him to grief and made Him sick" (The Amplified Bible).* If it was the will of God to bruise Him and make Him carry our sicknesses, how can it be the will of God to bruise us and make us carry those same sicknesses again? It can't be! That would be a travesty of divine justice!

If you want to see just how repulsive such a thought really is, switch things around for a moment. Think what your reaction would be if a fellow believer came to you and said, "Yesterday I got so drunk, I could hardly walk. Then I beat my wife and my kids. After that I robbed a gas station. But don't blame me for it. God put that sin on me to teach me something."

The very concept is revolting, isn't it? You would never tolerate it. You'd shut it down immediately. "Friend," you'd say, "you have the wrong idea. Jesus shed His precious blood to deliver you from sin. So if you choose to let it into your life, don't blame it on Him because it's not His fault!"

You may think that's an absurd example. You may think no one could ever be that foolish. But, the truth is, there were people in the Apostle Paul's day who preached that very thing. They went around saying that Paul's message of grace meant that we ought to sin so that grace could be shown.

That sounds silly to us today because we know that sin is repugnant to God. He hates it.

It's high time we realized that He hates sickness in the same way. Listen, sin, sickness and disease all came out of the same pit at the same time! God hates it when some devilish germ gnaws the life out of the body of one of His precious children. He designed and formed that body with His own hand out of the dust of the earth—and He made it perfect. How do you think He feels when He sees it twisted and tormented, bringing grief not only to the sufferer, but also to all those who love Him?

Don't you ever let anyone tell you that God likes that. He is a Father—not a monster! Such suffering could never be His will.

If by some convoluted stretch of the religious imagination we could decide it is His will for us to be sick, then we'll have to put the hospital and the beer joint in the same category. We'll have to condemn every doctor and every nurse for trying to thwart God's will.

"Now, Brother Copeland, that's stupid."

Yes, it is! Religious tradition is always stupid. It makes men believe things in church they'd never believe on the street. It makes them sit in a pew and agree with a preacher who says we learn from sickness and pain. "Oh yes, amen!" they'll say. But if that same preacher were to take a hammer, go down to the school and start knocking kids in the head to help them learn better, those same Amen-ers would have him arrested!

Healing Always Comes

Of course, some sincere-hearted believers have gotten confused about healing because they've seen or heard of instances where a good Christian didn't receive it. We've all heard the stories. "Well, healing couldn't be included in redemption because Sister So-and-So who taught Sunday school every week for 65 years got sick and God didn't heal her."

I want you to know something about those stories: They are lies. Granted, those who tell them usually don't realize it, but they are lies just the same.

I realize that's a shockingly blunt statement, but the Bible itself is just that blunt. It says: *"What if some did not believe and were without faith? Does their lack of faith and their faithlessness nullify and make ineffective and void the faithfulness of God and His fidelity [to His Word]? By no means! Let God be found true though every human being be false and a liar"* (Romans 3:3-4, *The Amplified Bible*).

God has made His Word plain to us. He has said, *"By His stripes we are healed"* (1 Peter 2:24). He has said, *"The prayer of faith shall save the sick, and the Lord shall raise him up"* (James 5:15). He has said, *"[Jesus] Himself took our infirmities, and bare our sicknesses"* (Matthew 8:17).

God always keeps His Word. Healing always comes. The problem has been in our receiving, not in God's giving.

Put that over in the realm of the new birth and you can easily see what I mean. The Bible says that by the righteousness of one, the free gift has come upon all men (Romans 5:18). Jesus has already gone to the cross and been raised from the dead. He has reconciled us to God and made righteousness available to every person on the face of the earth.

Therefore, it always comes. To whom? To anyone who will obey the instructions in

Romans 10:9-10: "...*if thou shalt confess with thy mouth the Lord Jesus, and shalt believe in thine heart that God hath raised him from the dead, thou shalt be saved. For with the heart man believeth unto righteousness; and with the mouth confession is made unto salvation.*"

Healing comes to the same people. It comes to those who will believe in their heart that Jesus was crucified and raised from the dead to purchase their healing. It comes to those who will open their mouths in faith and say, "Glory to God, I receive it. I am healed!"

Actually, if you could read that verse in the Greek, you'd see that it pertains to healing just as surely as to the new birth because the Greek word *sozo,* which is translated saved, literally means "to be made sound, to be delivered from every form of sickness and danger, both temporal and eternal."

What Do You Think Would Happen?

"But if receiving healing is as simple as receiving salvation," you ask, "why are so many Christians still sick?"

First and foremost, it's because the truth about healing has not been consistently preached. Since *"faith cometh by hearing, and hearing by the word of God"* (Romans 10:17), our failure to teach the fullness of the gospel has left many Christians without enough faith to heal a headache—much less cure cancer.

You know there was a time not so very long ago when it was just as tough to get people born again as it is to get them healed today. It's true! Religious tradition had convinced people that salvation just couldn't be obtained by the average person. But then, praise God, people like Dwight L. Moody came on the scene and started preaching the new birth. They started telling people that Jesus bore their sins and if they'd receive the gift of salvation in simple faith, they'd be born again!

Whole denominations like the Baptists preached that message to everything that would stand still. You'd hear it in every church service. If you walked in the door and admitted you weren't saved, somebody would grab you and say, "Jesus died for your sins, man! You don't have to stay in that condition. Just trust Him, receive Him as your Lord and He'll save you right now. Then He'll take you to heaven when you die!"

Praise God for all those precious Baptists and every other denomination like them! They preached the new birth until getting saved seemed like the easiest thing in the world.

Now what do you think would happen if everyone picked up on the truth about healing in that same way? What do you think would happen if every born-again believer in town started knocking on doors and having testimony meetings and revival meetings and telling everyone they meet a thousand times over, "Hey, man! Jesus bore your sicknesses and carried your diseases! You don't have to suffer with that cancer. Just trust Jesus and He'll heal you. He does it every time!"

I can tell you what would happen. Healing would become as common as the new birth and we'd wonder why we had so much trouble with it for so long!

What's more, in that environment, if someone prayed for healing and then said,

"I don't think I got anything. I don't feel any better," do you know what they'd be told? The same thing people are told today when they doubt their salvation because they don't "feel" saved.

Some mature believer would pull them aside and say, "Now listen, here. You can't go by feelings. You have to do this by faith. If you wait until you feel something to believe you're saved (or healed), you'll never be able to receive!"

Start Your Own Healing Revival

If you're sitting there right now wishing such a healing revival would begin, stop wishing and start your own! Dig into the Word. Study and meditate the truth about healing and redemption. Listen to tapes of men and women of God who have the revelation of it.

Then start preaching. Preach it to yourself. Preach it to your children. Preach it to your dog if he's the only one who will listen. It probably won't do much for him, but it will help you—and that's what matters.

If you'll do that, you'll eventually get to the point where you'll fight sickness and disease the same as you do sin. You'll be just as mean to Satan when it comes to standing for the redemption of your body as you are when it comes to the redemption of your spirit.

When he comes at you with symptoms of sickness, you won't crawl up in the bed and whine, "Why does this always happen to me?" You'll stomp your foot and say, "Glory be to God, this body is off limits to you, Satan. I refuse to allow you to put that foul thing on my body after Jesus has already borne it for me. So you might as well pack it up and go home right now!"

I'm not saying it will be easy. It won't be. Not in this life. Not in this world. Just as you don't live in victory over sin without putting forth an effort, you can't bumble along in life and have God just drop healing in your lap.

No, you'll have to stand for it. You'll have to fight the good fight of faith.

But don't let that scare you. It's a fight you can win. I know you can because 2,000 years ago, Jesus gave you everything you'd ever need to win it. He took your weakness and gave you His strength. He took your sin and gave you His righteousness. He took your sickness and gave you His health. He took your every defeat and gave you His victory in its place.

You are the heir of the Greatest Exchange ever made.

Begin to live like it and this world will never be the same again.

God's Prescription for Divine Health

"My son, attend to my words; incline thine ear unto my sayings. Let them not depart from thine eyes; keep them in the midst of thine heart. For they are life unto those that find them, and health to all their flesh. Keep thy heart with all diligence; for out of it are the issues of life. Put away from thee a froward mouth, and perverse lips put far from thee."
— PROVERBS 4:20-24

Gloria Copeland

There is a medicine so powerful it can cure every sickness and disease known to man. It has no dangerous side effects. It is safe even in massive doses. And when taken daily according to directions, it can prevent illness altogether and keep you in vibrant health.

Does that sound too good to be true? It's not. I can testify to you by the Word of God and by my own experience that such a supernatural medicine exists. Even more importantly, it is available to you every moment of every day.

You don't have to call your doctor to get it. You don't even have to drive to the pharmacy. All you must do is reach for your Bible, open to Proverbs 4:20-24 and follow the instructions you find there: *"My son, attend to my words; incline thine ear unto my sayings. Let them not depart from thine eyes; keep them in the midst of thine heart. For they are life unto those that find them, and health [Hebrew: medicine] to all their flesh. Keep thy heart with all diligence; for out of it are the issues of life. Put away from thee a froward mouth, and perverse lips put far from thee."*

As simple as they might sound, those four verses contain the supernatural prescription to divine health. It's a powerful prescription that will work for anyone who will put it to work.

If you have received healing by the laying on of hands, following this prescription will help you maintain that healing. If you have believed for healing, but are experiencing lingering symptoms, it will help you stand strong until you are completely symptom-free. And if you are healthy now, it will help you stay that way—not just for a day or a week, but for the rest of your life!

Powerful Medicine

To understand how this prescription works, you must realize that the Word of God is more than just good information. It actually has life in it. As Jesus said in John 6:63, *"It is the spirit that quickeneth [or makes alive]; the flesh profiteth nothing: the words that I speak unto you, they are spirit, and they are life."*

Every time you take the Word into your heart, believe it and act on it, that life of which Jesus spoke, the very LIFE of God Himself, is released in you. You may have read the healing scriptures over and over again. You may know them as well as you know your own name. Yet every time you read them or hear them preached, they bring you a fresh dose of God's healing power. Each time, they bring life to you and deliver God's medicine to your flesh.

That's because the Word is like a seed. Hebrews 4:12 says it is *"alive and full of power—making it active, operative, energizing and effective..." (The Amplified Bible).* It actually carries within it the power to fulfill itself.

When you planted the Word about the new birth in your heart, then believed and acted on it, that Word released within you the power to be born again. By the same token, when you plant the Word about healing in your heart, believe and act on it, that Word will release God's healing power in you.

"But, Gloria," you may say, "I've met people who know the Bible from cover to cover and still can't get healed!"

No doubt you do. But if you'll look back at God's prescription, you'll find it doesn't say anything about "knowing" the Bible. It says, attend to the Word.

When you attend to something, you give your attention to it. You make it top priority. You set aside other things so you can focus on it. When a nurse is attending to a patient, she constantly looks after him. She doesn't just leave him lying alone in his hospital room while she goes shopping. If someone asks her about her patient, she doesn't feel it's sufficient to say, "Oh, yes. I know him."

In the same way, if you're attending to the Word, you won't leave it lying unopened on the coffee table all day. You won't spend your day focusing your attention on other things.

On the contrary, you'll do what Proverbs 4 says to do. You'll continually incline your ear to God's Word.

Inclining your ear includes more than just putting your physical ears in a position to hear the Word being preached (although that, in itself, is very important). It also requires you to actively engage with God's Word, to believe it and obey it.

In fact, *The Amplified Bible* translates Proverbs 4:20, this way: *"My son, attend to my words; consent and submit to my sayings."* Submitting to the Word means making adjustments in your life. Say, for example, you hear the Word in Philippians 4:4 that you are to *"rejoice in the Lord always."* If you've been doing a lot of griping and complaining, you'll have to change in order to submit to that Word. You'll have to repent and alter your behavior.

Take as Directed

In addition to inclining your ear to the Word of God, the Proverbs 4 prescription also says you must keep it before your eyes and not let it depart from your sight. In Matthew 6:22-23, Jesus reveals why that's so important. He says, *"The light of the body is the eye: if therefore thine eye be single, thy whole body shall be full of light. But if thine eye be evil, thy whole body shall be full of darkness. If therefore the light that is in thee be darkness, how great is that darkness!"*

Your eyes are the gateway to your body. If your eye (or your attention) is on the darkness, or the sickness that is in your body, there will be no light to expel it. If, however, the eyes of your heart are trained strictly on the

Word, your whole body will eventually be filled with light, and healing will be the result.

Granted, it isn't easy to keep your attention centered on the Word like that. It takes real effort and commitment. It may require getting up a little earlier in the morning or turning off the television at night. But I urge you to do whatever it takes to take God's medicine exactly as directed.

It won't work any other way!

That really shouldn't be so surprising. After all, we wouldn't expect natural medication to work for us if we didn't take it as prescribed.

No rational person would set a bottle of pills on the night stand and expect those pills to heal them. No one would call the doctor and say, "Hey, Doc! These pills don't work. I've carried them with me everywhere I go—I keep them in the car with me, I set them on my desk at work, I even have them next to me when I sleep at night—but I don't feel any better."

That would be ridiculous. Yet, spiritually speaking, some people do it all the time. They cry and pray and beg God to heal them, all the while ignoring the medicine He's provided. (They might take a quick dose on Sunday when they go to church, but the rest of the week they don't take time for the Word at all!)

Why do people who love God and believe the Bible act that way? I think it's because they don't understand how putting the Word in their heart can affect their physical bodies. They don't see how something spiritual can change something natural.

If you'll read the Bible, however, you'll see that spiritual power has been affecting this physical world ever since time began. In fact, it was spiritual power released in the form of God's Word that brought this natural world into existence in the first place.

When you realize that God's Word is the force that originally brought into being everything you can see and touch—including your physical body—it's easy to believe that the Word is still capable of changing your body today. It makes perfect sense!

Faith in Two Places

"I'd have no problem at all believing God's Word would heal me if He'd speak to me out loud like He did in Genesis," you might say, "but He hasn't!"

No, and He probably won't either. God no longer has to thunder His Word down at us from heaven. These days He lives in the hearts of believers, so He speaks to us from the inside instead of the outside. What's more, when it comes to covenant issues like healing, we don't even have to wait on Him to speak.

He has already spoken!

He has already said, *"By [Jesus'] stripes ye were healed"* (1 Peter 2:24). He has already said, *"I am the Lord that healeth thee"* (Exodus 15:26). He has already said, *"The prayer of faith shall save the sick, and the Lord shall raise him up"* (James 5:15).

God has already done His part. So we must do ours. We must take the Word He has spoken, put it inside us and let it change us from the inside out.

You see, everything—including healing—starts inside you. Your future is literally stored up in your heart. As Jesus said, *"A good man out of the good treasure of the heart bringeth forth good things: and an evil man out of the evil treasure bringeth forth evil things"* (Matthew 12:35).

That means if you want external conditions to be better tomorrow, you'd better start changing your internal condition today. You'd better start taking the Word of God and depositing it in your heart just like you deposit money in the bank. Then you can make withdrawals on it whenever you need it. When sickness attacks your body, you can tap into the healing Word you've put inside you and run that sickness off!

Exactly how do you do that?

You open your mouth and speak—not words of sickness and disease, discouragement and despair, but words of healing and life, faith and hope. You follow the last step of God's divine prescription and *"Put away from thee a froward mouth, and perverse lips put far from thee"* (Proverbs 4:24). In short, you speak the words of God and call yourself healed in Jesus' Name.

Initially, that may not be easy for you to do. But you must do it anyway because for faith to work it must be in two places—in your heart and in your mouth. *"For with the heart man believeth unto righteousness; and with the mouth confession is made unto salvation"* (Romans 10:10).

Some people say faith will move mountains. But, the scriptural truth is, faith won't even move a molehill for you unless you release it with the words of your mouth.

The Lord Jesus told us that *"...whosoever shall say unto this mountain, Be thou removed, and be thou cast into the sea; and shall not doubt in his heart, but shall believe that those things which he saith shall come to pass; he shall have whatsoever he saith"* (Mark 11:23). Notice the word *say* appears three times in that verse while the word *believe* appears only once. Obviously, Jesus wanted us to know that our words are crucial.

It's also important to note that He did not instruct us to talk about the mountain, He instructed us to talk to it! If we're going to obey Him, we must talk to the mountain of sickness and cast it out of our lives. The Lord told Charles Capps, *I have told My people they can have what they say, but they are saying what they have!* Instead of saying, "I'm healed," most Christians say, "I'm sick," and reinforce the sickness or disease.

"But, Gloria, it bothers me to say I'm healed when my body still feels sick!"

It shouldn't. It didn't bother Abraham. He went around calling himself the Father of Nations for years even though he was as childless as could be. Why did he do it? Because *"he believed...God, who quickeneth the dead, and calleth those things which be not as though they were"* (Romans 4:17). He was *"fully persuaded that, what [God] had promised, he was able also to perform"* (verse 21).

You see, Abraham wasn't "trying" to believe God. He wasn't just mentally assenting to it. He had immersed himself in God's Word until that Word was more real to him than the things he could see. It didn't matter to him that he was 100 years old. It didn't matter to him that Sarah was far past the age of childbearing and that she had been barren all her life. All that mattered to him was what God said, because he knew His Word was true.

If you don't have that kind of faith for healing right now, then stay in the Word until you get it! After all, *"faith cometh by hearing, and hearing by the word of God"* (Romans 10:17). Read, study, meditate, listen to tapes, watch videos of good, faith-filled teaching, and watch our Sunday and daily television broadcast EVERY DAY until God's Word about healing is more real to you than the symptoms in your body. Keep on keeping on until, like Abraham, you "stagger not at the promise of God through unbelief, but grow strong in faith as you give praise and glory to God." (See Romans 4:20, *The Amplified Bible*).

Having Done All...Stand!

As you put God's prescription for health to work in your life, don't be discouraged if you don't see immediate results. Although many times healing comes instantly, there also are times when it takes place more gradually.

So don't let lingering symptoms cause you to doubt. After all, when you go to the doctor, you don't always feel better right away. The medication he gives you often takes some time before it begins to work. But you don't allow the delay to discourage you. You just follow the doctor's orders and expect to feel better soon. Really, you are "treating" your spirit, which is the source of supernatural life and health for your physical body.

Release that same kind of confidence in God's medicine. Realize that the moment you begin to take it, the healing process begins. Keep your expectancy high and make up your mind to continue standing on the Word until you can see and feel the total physical effects of God's healing power.

When the devil whispers words of doubt and unbelief to you, when he suggests that the Word is not working, deal with those thoughts immediately. Cast them down (see 2 Corinthians 10:5). Speak out loud if necessary and say, "Devil, I rebuke you. I bind you from my mind. I will not believe your lies. God has sent His Word to heal me, and His Word never fails. That Word went to work in my body the instant I believed it, so as far as I am concerned, my days of sickness are over. I declare that Jesus bore my sickness, weakness and pain, and I am forever free."

Then, *"having done all, to stand. Stand"* until your healing is fully manifested (see Ephesians 6:12-14). Steadfastly hold your ground. Don't waver. For as James 1:6-8 says, *"...He that wavereth is like a wave of the sea driven with the wind and tossed.... Let not that man think that he shall receive any thing of the Lord. A double minded man is unstable in all his ways."*

Above all, keep your attention trained on the Word—not on lingering symptoms. Be like Abraham who *"considered not his own body"* (Romans 4:19). Instead of focusing on your circumstances, focus on what God has said to you. Develop an inner image of yourself with your healing fully manifested. See yourself well. See yourself whole. See yourself healed in every way.

Since what you keep before your eyes and in your ears determines what you will believe in your heart and what you will act on, make the Word your number one priority. Keep taking God's medicine as directed and trust the Great Physician to do His wonderful healing work in you!

More Than a New Year's Resolution

"Commit thy way unto the LORD; trust also in him; and he shall bring it to pass."
— PSALM 37:5

Marty Copeland

At the same time every year many people make New Year's resolutions. For most, these resolutions are earnest attempts to change. Unfortunately, most people don't realize they're setting themselves up for failure.

A New Year's resolution promises gain, but lacks the substance to produce it. Any resolution that tries to bring about a transformation by fleshly effort instead of by the power of God sets you up for failure. It has no substance.

Lasting victory is never won by our own might or power. True change and total victory occur only when we exercise our faith in the transforming power of God alone.

As a certified personal trainer and aerobics instructor, I'm regularly involved with people who battle overeating or other compulsive behaviors. In their determination to break free from the grip of destructive habits, they often make desperate resolutions. My heart goes out to them because I used to be trapped in that same struggle. For over half my life, I was in bondage to overeating. I was obsessed with diets and exercise. I lost close to a total of 700 pounds through years of gaining, then losing weight. Today, I'm totally, 100 percent free and experiencing the joy that comes with that freedom. But there was a time when I, like so many others, began each New Year with noble resolutions. I always hoped that this year my resolution would be "The Solution"—only to find myself failing and feeling miserable...again.

In theory, resolutions sound good. In practice, however, they fall short. Desperate resolutions are just carnal methods that play right into Satan's deceptive strategy to keep us frustrated and failing until finally we lose all hope that we'll ever be free.

If Satan can keep you in the arena of the flesh, using carnal weapons to fight a spiritual warfare, he can defeat you. But if you'll take the weapons of your warfare which are not carnal but mighty through God, you can defeat the devil and overcome destructive habits in every area of your life.

Jesus said if we continue in His Word, we shall know the truth and the truth shall make us free (John 8:31-32). So don't let the devil lure you into another cycle of failure and disappointment with the temptation of a "quick fix." There is a way out. But you'll need more than a New Year's resolution—you'll need to make a quality decision to put your hope and faith in God.

As you continue in the Word and trust God to conform you to the image of His Son, that burden-removing, yoke-destroying power of Jesus the Anointed One and His anointing will set you free from the bondage of weight and the weight of bondage. You can confidently put your hope and trust in Him because when the Son makes you free, you are free indeed (John 8:36)!

Harvest of Health

"So shall my word be that goeth forth out of my mouth: it shall not return unto me void, but it shall accomplish that which I please, and it shall prosper in the thing whereto I sent it."
— ISAIAH 55:11

Gloria
Copeland

I have some revolutionary news for you. God wants you healthy! Every day!

Oh, I know that, you may quickly think, *I know God will heal me when I get sick.*

Yes, that's true, He will. But that's not what I'm saying. I'm telling you God's perfect will is for you to live continually in divine health. His will is for you to walk so fully in the power of His Word that sickness and disease are literally pushed away from you. Isn't that good news?

You've probably heard a lot about God's healing power but there is a difference between divine healing and divine health.

Years ago, the powerful preacher John G. Lake put it this way, "Divine healing is the removal by the power of God of the disease that has come upon the body. But divine health is to live day by day, hour by hour in touch with God so that the life of God flows into the body just as the life of God flows into the mind or flows into the spirit."

I agree that it is wonderful to get healed when you're sick, but it's more wonderful to live in divine health. And that's what God has always intended for His people. Even under the Old Covenant God promised His people immunity from disease. Exodus 23:25 says, *"And ye shall serve the Lord your God, and he shall bless thy bread, and thy water; and I will take sickness away from the midst of thee."*

That promise is even stronger under the New Covenant. Isaiah, looking forward to what Jesus would accomplish on the cross wrote, *"Surely he [Jesus] hath borne our griefs, and carried our sorrows...he was wounded for our transgressions, he was bruised for our iniquities: the chastisement of our peace was upon him; and with his stripes we are healed"* (Isaiah 53:4-5).

The Apostle Peter, looking back at that same event wrote, *"Who his own self bare our sins in his own body on the tree, that we, being dead to sins, should live unto righteousness: by whose stripes ye were healed"* (1 Peter 2:24).

"Were healed!" That's past tense. Jesus finished your healing on the cross. He paid the price for you to be whole. He bought righteousness for your spirit, peace for your mind and healing for your body.

As far as Jesus is concerned, you're not the sick trying to get healed. You're the healed and Satan is trying to steal your health. I remember when Ken and I realized that, it changed everything for us. We quit trying to talk God into healing us and began instead resisting sickness and disease the way we resisted sin.

No Third Story on a Vacant Lot

Once you understand God's will really is for you to live in divine health, you can't help but question why so many believers live sick. It seems puzzling at first. But the answer is very simple. Many of them just aren't willing to do what it takes to be well.

People want to be well. No one wants to be sick. But to be well, you have to make choices. How often have you seen someone with a hacking cough still smoking a cigarette? Or an overweight person eating an ice cream cone?

Our fleshly nature likes to take the easy way. And it's much easier to give in to habits than to break them. It's easier to give in to your flesh and watch television every night like the rest of the world, than to spend your time putting God's healing Word into your heart.

I recently heard Charles Capps say that some people try to build the third story of a building on a vacant lot. That sounds funny, but spiritually speaking it's true. A lot of people want to enjoy the benefits of healing without building the foundation for it from the Word of God.

It can't be done. If you want a building, you have to start below ground level. If you want a harvest, you're going to have to plant something first.

Everything in the natural world works that way. Ken calls it the law of genesis. This law of planting and reaping works in the spirit realm too. It governs health, prosperity—in fact, everything in God's kingdom is governed by the law of planting and reaping.

Jesus taught about it in Mark 4:26-29. There, He said:

> **So is the kingdom of God, as if a man should cast seed into the ground; And should sleep, and rise night and day, and the seed should spring and grow up, he knoweth not how. For the earth bringeth forth fruit of herself; first the blade, then the ear, after that the full corn in the ear. But when the fruit is brought forth, immediately he putteth in the sickle, because the harvest is come.**

According to the law of sowing and reaping, if you want health, you need to do more than just want it. You even need to do more than believe in healing. You need to plant seed that will eventually grow up and yield a harvest of health.

What kind of seed produces physical health? Proverbs 4:20-22 tells us: *"My son, attend to my words; incline thine ear unto my sayings. Let them not depart from thine eyes; keep them in the midst of thine heart. For they are life unto those that find them, and health to all their flesh."*

That word *health* in Hebrew means "medicine." God's Word has life in it. It is actually spirit food. As you feed on it, you become strong spiritually and physically.

"Let them not depart from thine eyes...." Read the Word. Meditate on the Word. That's taking God's medicine. If you will be faithful to take it continually, it eventually will be as hard for you to get sick as it ever was for you to get well.

But it's a process. You can't just read the healing scriptures once and then go on about your business. You must continually feed on the Word of God to keep the crop of healing coming up in your life.

What Did You Say?

Isaiah 55:11 says the Word of God prospers (or succeeds) in the thing for which it is sent. That means His Word about healing will produce healing. It may not produce it right away, but the more you let the Word work in you, the greater your results will be.

In other words, the size of your harvest will depend on how much seed you plant. How much time and attention you give to the Word of God will determine how much crop you will yield.

You see, your heart is actually your spirit. Its capacity is unlimited. You can plant as much seed in your heart as you have hours in a day.

If you'll build your life around the Word, you can have a full return. Jesus called it a hundredfold return (Mark 4:20).

Now some people will argue about that. They'll say, "Well, it didn't work for me! I put God's Word about healing into my heart and I'm still sick!"

But do you know what? They give themselves away the minute they say such things. Jesus taught, *"Out of the abundance of the heart the mouth speaketh"* (Matthew 12:34). If those people had actually planted God's Word in their hearts in abundance, they'd be talking about healing, not sickness! They would be saying, "By His stripes I am healed!"

The same is true for you. The more you put God's Word in your heart, the stronger you'll become. And eventually that Word inside you will begin to come out of your mouth in power and deliverance.

Don't wait until you have a need to start speaking the Word. Start speaking it now.

I'll never forget the first time I realized the importance of speaking God's Word. It was years ago when Ken had just started preaching and I was staying at home with our children. We were in a desperate situation financially and I was eager for answers.

One day as I was sitting at my typewriter, typing notes and listening to tapes, I read Mark 11:23. *"For verily I say unto you, That whosoever shall say unto this mountain, Be thou removed, and be thou cast into the sea; and shall not doubt in his heart, but shall believe that those things which he saith shall come to pass; he shall have whatsoever he saith."*

Suddenly, the truth of that last phrase just jumped out at me. And the Lord spoke to my heart and said, *In consistency lies the power.*

He was telling me that it's not just the words you speak when you pray that change things, it's the words you speak all the time!

If you want to see your desire come to pass, you need to make your words match your prayers. Don't try to pray in faith and then get up and talk unbelief. Talk faith all the time!

Romans 4:17 says God *"calleth those things which be not as though they were."* So if you want to receive something from God, follow His example. Speak it. That's the way faith works. You speak the Word of God concerning what you want to happen.

If what you're looking for is health, then go to the Word that tells you, "By His stripes you were healed," and put that in your mouth. Don't talk sickness. Talk health. Don't talk the problem. Talk the answer.

What You Plant Always Grows

"But Gloria," you say, "all that sounds so simple!"

It is simple! Sometimes I think that's why God chose me to teach it. Because I'm simple. When I read the Word of God, I just believe it is speaking to me personally. I don't worry and fuss and say, "Well, I wish that would work for me, but I don't think it will because of this or that...." I just expect God to do what He says.

You can do the same thing. You can come to the Word like a little child and say, "Lord, I receive this. I believe Your Word above all and I trust You with my life." If you will, you'll never be disappointed.

How can you get that kind of simple, childlike faith? By hearing the Word of God.

Romans 10:17 says, *"faith cometh by hearing, and hearing by the word of God."* But you need to know something else: Doubt comes by hearing also. That's why Jesus said, *"Be careful what you are hearing..."* (Mark 4:24, *The Amplified Bible*).

What you're hearing can be a matter of life and death when you're dealing with healing. If you're going to a church, for example, that teaches healing has passed away or that God uses sickness to teach you something—and you keep hearing that Sunday after Sunday—what do you think will grow in your heart? Doubt, not faith.

What you plant inside your heart grows— always. Doubt will grow and keep you bound. Truth will grow and make you free. So be careful what you're hearing. Listen to the Word of God. As Proverbs 4:21 says, *"Let them [that Word] not depart from thine eyes; keep them [it] in the midst of thine heart."*

Read the Word every day. Make note cards for yourself using the healing scriptures and tape them to your mirror.

Play teaching tapes. Listen to them in your car. Listen to them while you dress in the morning. If you'll listen to the Word while you're driving back and forth to work every day, you'll be surprised how fruitful that time will become. It will change your life. I challenge you to try it!

Don't Let Them Throw You

God's words have power in them. When you keep them in the midst of your heart, they become life and healing and health. They're medicine. God's medicine.

But beware. People will try to discourage you and keep you from taking that medicine. They'll tell you things like, "If God wants us to live in divine health, why did Sister So-and-So suffer so much sickness? And she was a fine Christian."

Don't let them throw you off track. Instead, just remember this: You don't live in divine health because you're a fine Christian. No one does. You live in divine health because you take the Word of God, and you keep it in front of your eyes. You keep it going in your ears. You keep it in the midst of your heart and you apply it to your life.

You live in divine health because you believe God for it, because you talk about it, and because you act on it—day, after day, after day.

Don't wait until an emergency comes. Don't wait until your body is weak and sick to start feeding on healing scriptures. Start now. Plant God's Word of healing in the good faith-soil of your heart daily—and then, get excited. Your harvest of health is on its way!

Chapter 5

Stop Those Fits of Carnality!

"To be carnally minded is death; but to be spiritually minded is life and peace."
— ROMANS 8:6

My blood was boiling!

There I was on my way to a spiritual meeting. Born again, Spirit filled and anointed of God for ministry—I was on a mission and late for my plane. With my wife Cathy in the passenger seat and our 6-year-old daughter in the back, I had been making good time.

Then another car came flying out on the road. From a fast rate of 60 miles an hour, the car slowed to 35. I tried to pass, but the driver thought both lanes belonged to her. You've probably been behind a man or woman who drove like that. I went to the left—she went to the left. I went to the right—she went to the right.

Soon Tabasco™ sauce was coming up my legs: "God, DO something with this woman!"

I began to shout through the windshield to her. "Hey, if you can't drive the car, park it!" Finally, I thought, *Brother, if she just goes to the right a half inch, I'm going to put my foot in the carburetor, slam to the left, hit the grass, ride the median—whatever—I'm going to pass that woman!*

I fussed. I fumed. But before I got my chance to pass her, the muffler fell off her car. I was too close to miss it. Boom, boom, boom, boom, boom. Two of my tires were destroyed.

As she puttered off across the horizon, I shouted, "Why you...if I could catch you...."

Then out of the mouth of babes....

"You'd tell her that Jesus loves her, huh, Daddy?" my daughter interrupted.

What had I done?

I had a fit—a fit of carnality.

Had Any Fits Lately?

You've had your fits, too. Don't try to tell me you haven't!

It may have happened after you watched a dessert commercial on television—and before you knew it you were in the kitchen stuffing cake in your mouth as fast as you could. It may have happened when an anointed church service went past lunch. It may have happened with someone you love—one day you were saying, "I love my wife so much. I can't live without her." The next day you were saying, "How'd we get together? Get out of my way!"

These are fits of carnality—fits where you let your flesh take over. Jesus knew what they were. Paul knew too. He'd had his share. In Romans 8:6-8 he tells us very clearly about fits of carnality: *"For to be carnally minded is death; but to be spiritually minded is life and peace. Because the carnal mind is enmity against God: for it is not subject to the law of God, neither indeed can be. So then they that are in the flesh cannot please God."*

What was Paul saying? That "your fits of carnality have almost cost you your life." Any time we get out of the realm of faith, we get into the realm of carnality, or flesh and death. We get into a realm where we cannot please God, because without faith it is impossible to please God (Hebrews 11:6). Any time we get out of faith and into the carnal realm, we have set ourselves up for a fit of carnality.

A Dead Cat and a Disobedient Woman!

Soon after I was saved, the pipes froze and broke on our little house in Southern Louisiana. I had been a rock musician, not a handyman, so I was not looking forward to this chore. I pulled on my coveralls and dragged myself through a sea of cold water and mud in 30-degree weather. I was aggravated, uncomfortable and needed a helper.

So I asked Cathy, "Cathy, I need some help."

"Oh, I can't come underneath that house," she said. "There's spiders under there."

That made me so mad. "I NEED SOME HELP!"

"I can't crawl underneath that house....
It's dirty," she said. "But I'll help you."

How? I wondered.

"All right," I said, but I just got madder.
Then I cut myself on a piece of broken
glass. And I busted my knuckles trying to
break the old piece of pipe out. But finally,
I got the cold line fixed.

"Cathy," I hollered through the floor,
"there's two knobs, one on the left and one
on the right. Don't touch the left knob.
That's the hot water. Turn on the right knob,
because the cold line's fixed."

"OK."

An instant later I was being scalded with
hot water. She had turned on the left knob!

"Cathy, turn it off. I am being burned!"

Cathy turned it off, and came to apolo-
gize. As she looked down under the house,
she said, "Oh, Jesse, don't move! There's a
dead cat by your head."

I had smelled a strange odor, but only then
did I see it—a cat with its brains hanging out.

"GRAB IT!" I told her.

"I don't touch dead cats," she squealed.

And then I had a fit.

"Woman, when I get out from under this house...."

As I pushed the cat, a thorn jabbed me in the back.

"What is this?" I wailed.

"Oh, I threw some cactus underneath the house," Cathy said.

Cactus...dead cat...scalding water. Did I ever have a fit of carnality. With cuts in my body and a cat in my hand, I was tearing out from underneath that house ready to tell Cathy what I thought when I was greeted by my unsaved neighbor.

"How you doing, preacher?" he asked. "You know I wouldn't touch that dead cat if I were you. What's the problem anyway?"

I'd been witnessing to this man. Suddenly, I didn't know what to say. But he surmised things pretty quickly.

"Your wife won't help you, huh?"

I said, "How'd you know that?"

"Well, I busted a pipe earlier this morning and tried to get my wife to help. She wouldn't do it either. You want me to give you a hand?"

While I'd been telling this man "Jesus is the greatest thing in the world. My God gives. Jesus can handle anything..." my actions were adding...except a broken pipe and a dead cat and a disobedient woman!

You can take this to the bank: Every time you have a fit of carnality, somebody is going to see you do it. So how do we stop ourselves from having these fits?

Sound Words Are Salvation Words

First, do what Paul told Timothy to do: *"Hold fast the form of sound words, which thou hast heard of me, in faith and love which is in Christ Jesus. That good thing which was committed unto thee keep by the Holy Ghost which dwelleth in us"* (2 Timothy 1:13-14).

That day, years ago, as I was driving to the airport, I had a choice. I could have

71

prayed this: "Lord, I'm kind of in a hurry. Would You mind moving that little lady over to the side?"

But it seemed like it was much easier to holler through the windshield. I didn't hold fast to the form of sound words. Instead, I gave myself over to "no" words—words that had no power to bring God on the scene of my need.

Sound words are salvation words. They are the words that can change your situation. They are words that feed and strengthen your spirit.

You will not overcome fits of carnality by focusing your efforts on the flesh. There's no good thing in the flesh. If you think in your finite mind that you're going get this flesh to become holy, you have missed it by 100 miles. First Corinthians 2:14 tells us that *"the natural man receiveth not the things of the Spirit of God: for they are foolishness unto him: neither can he know them, because they are spiritually discerned."*

But if you will feed and strengthen your spirit on sound words, you will become no longer conformed to this world, but transformed by the renewing of your mind (Romans 12:2). Sound words will turn your spirit into a dynamo that totally regenerates the thought processes of your soul (mind, will and emotions). And then from that mind, will and emotion (soul) will come a cross that crucifies your flesh on a daily basis. If the weight of the Cross is on your mind, will and emotions, you will speak words of faith. Any time you are speaking soundly, a fit will not take place.

Submit Yourself to God

Second, when you see a fit of carnality coming on, *"Submit yourselves therefore to God. Resist the devil, and he will flee from you"* (James 4:7). What we typically want to do first is to deal more with our anger than with our submitting. We want to start rebuking the devil. But that's the wrong order. Before the devil is ever mentioned, before we have our full-blown fit of carnality, we must first submit ourselves to God.

To submit to God, we must first know what God has said. If we know what He has said, then we should be repeating what He has said. We should speak sound words, and submit ourselves to what we are speaking.

The Bible prophet Elijah spoke God's Word boldly in the presence of the people, challenging the prophets of Baal. When he did, God confirmed those words with a mighty demonstration of His power.

Then Queen Jezebel threatened to kill him, and Elijah took off running. He had a fit of carnality. Why? Because he didn't submit to the sound words that he was speaking about God's power to deliver. Elijah's first thought was that Jezebel was more powerful than he. Eventually, he realized what he had done and did submit to God's Word.

So say what God has said, then make sure you submit to the sound words you are saying. You may be saying and believing the right things, but if you don't submit yourself to what you believe, you'll have a fit of carnality every day of your life.

Resist (Don't Assist) the Devil

Finally, resist the devil. Notice the order in James 4:7, *"Submit yourselves therefore to God. Resist the devil, and he will flee from you."* First submit to God, then resist the devil.

For years I didn't know how to resist the devil. I blamed my temper on my Cajun heritage. Finally the Lord said, *Jesse, it's just you assisting the devil!*

As long as we are assisting the devil instead of resisting him, he's going to be running toward us and not away from us. We'll actually just be helping him with our fits of carnality.

Peter was known for fits like this. When the priests and soldiers came to arrest Jesus, Peter pulled out a knife and cut a guy's ear off. Just ripped it off, thinking he was helping.

Jesus picked the guy's ear up and put it back on his head, saying, "What's the matter with you, Peter?"

Peter was probably thinking: *I was just trying to help You out.*

You can be sitting in a meeting where there is a mighty move of God and be having a fit of carnality because you have not submitted yourself to God, and have not resisted the devil. Maybe your body is rebelling because the service is going so long. Or you may be embarrassed because under the anointing your wife seems out of control. You're assisting the devil, and you can grieve the Holy Ghost right in the middle of a powerful service. Someone may not get saved or healed because you had a fit of carnality.

Many of us are like Peter—we need time to grow. And the way we grow is by submitting ourselves to God. Then we can begin to resist the devil instead of assisting him. Soon we'll find Satan beginning to flee from us instead of coming toward us, and our fits of carnality will happen less and less.

Watch the Devil Run!

Don't misunderstand me. I'm not saying this life is easy. Everyone has aggravations. But an aggravation does not have to grow into a full-blown, no-holds-barred fit of carnality.

Hold fast to the form of sound words which you've heard of God. Live as a child of God, led by the Spirit of God, and submitted to Him. *"For as many as are led by the Spirit of God, they are the sons of God"* (Romans 8:14). You can walk in the spirit—all the time. The promise of that walk is life and peace (see Romans 8:6).

As you allow yourself to be led by the Spirit, He will give you opportunity to take authority over that aggravation so that it doesn't become a fit of carnality. Soon you'll be resisting the devil instead of assisting him.

Satan always works through a fit of carnality. If you will jump this hurdle and take away his ability to work up a fit of carnality in you, you will have closed the door to almost anything he could ever do to you. And whenever you're around, all he'll have left to do is to turn his tail and run!

Winning the Battle of the Flesh

"For though we walk in the flesh, we do not war after the flesh: (For the weapons of our warfare are not carnal, but mighty through God to the pulling down of strong holds;) Casting down imaginations, and every high thing that exalteth itself against the knowledge of God, and bringing into captivity every thought to the obedience of Christ."
— 2 Corinthians 10:3-5

Kenneth Copeland

Do you know what it's like to be in a losing battle with your own body? I do... and I can tell you, it's miserable.

There have been times in my life as a believer when I wanted with all my heart to behave one way, and my body seemed absolutely intent on doing exactly the opposite. Times when I desperately wanted to lose excess weight, yet kept right on stuffing myself with every kind of unhealthy food I could get my hands on. Times, years ago, when I so longed to quit smoking that I threw my cigarettes out the car window... then turned the car around to go back and get them when I realized I didn't have the money for another pack.

You know what I'm talking about. You've been there too. Every Christian has in one way or another. We call it the battle of the flesh.

The crucial element in having victory is making a quality decision, one from which there is no retreat and about which there is no argument. It is the one thing God will not do for you. He has set before us life and death, but the actual choosing, the quality decision, is up to you.

But once you've made that quality decision, how do you stand when your flesh moans and groans and kicks and fusses? When you feel torn in two? When you're tempted to condemn yourself?

You take authority over your flesh—and you win.

Some people would say, "Oh yes, Brother Copeland. We have to fight our flesh constantly. It has an evil nature, the nature of the old man, you know, and it opposes the nature of God in us."

Please excuse me for being blunt, but I have to tell you, that's the most schizophrenic thing I've ever heard in my life. When we're born again, we're not half God and half devil. Jesus paid the price for our whole being on the Cross—spirit, soul and body.

It bothers me when I hear a believer talk about his old, wicked, sinful, terrible flesh. We shouldn't talk like that! Jesus allowed stripes to be laid on His back so that our flesh could be healed. Ephesians 5:29 says, *"...no man ever yet hated his own flesh; but nourisheth and cherisheth it...."* You're doing something that is unscriptural and unnatural in the sight of God when you begin to hate your own body.

"But I thought we were supposed to crucify our flesh!"

If you're born again, you've already done that. Galatians 5:24 says, *"And they that are Christ's have crucified the flesh with the affections and lusts."*

"Then why am I still having such a struggle?"

Quite simply, it's because you haven't developed your ability to walk in the Spirit. For as Galatians 5:16 says, if you *walk in the Spirit...ye shall not fulfil the lust of the flesh.* It does not say, "Hate your flesh enough, and someday maybe it will settle down."

Flesh Does What It's Told

To fully understand what I'm saying, there are some things you need to understand about your physical body. Number one is the fact that it has no nature of its own. It's just flesh, blood and bone that does what it has been trained to do.

Simply put, your flesh does what it's told to do. For example, if you decide to stand up, your body will stand up, right? But has your body ever just jumped up and run all around on its own without consulting you? Of course not! It's not made to do that.

Now once you train your body and teach it to do certain things and act in certain ways, it will expand and develop in those abilities. It will actually begin to do those things without conscious thought on your part. If it weren't that way, you'd still be struggling trying to button your shirt for 20 minutes like you did when you were four years old. You'd never be able to expand in any direction if your body couldn't accept training.

The problem most believers have with their flesh is that it's still living the way they trained it to live before they were born again. It's trying to go that same old sinful way it has practiced for so many years. It doesn't yet know the believer has been saved.

What's more, it's being successful in going that way because instead of taking charge of their flesh and putting it under the direction of their spirit, those believers have let their flesh run the show.

Let me tell you, that's backward. Your flesh has no business lording over your spirit. It does not have the equipment, the ability, the calling, or the nature to rule this human system. It is merely a tool. It is a natural vehicle that enables the spirit man to live and have authority in this natural, physical world.

The body is not equipped to be in charge. Neither is the mind. When leadership pressure is put on the mind, eventually it will snap.

That's why it is so vital to understand that you are a spirit, you have a soul and you live in a body. Your spirit man, once it's been born again and re-created by the Spirit of God, is equipped to rule that system. A reborn spirit man has the capacity to take the mental computer God gave him and the body God put him in and bring them both into obedience to Christ Jesus. The spirit man is equipped for ascendancy over the human system. When he's in charge, taught and trained by the Holy Spirit and infused with power from on high, he simply cannot be beaten!

But far too many believers are living backward. They're allowing their bodies, which are highly skilled and trained in the ways of the world, to determine their choices in life. They know they shouldn't—and they struggle against it by trying to impose external rules and regulations on themselves. But that doesn't work. You can't train the flesh from the outside in; you have to do it from the inside out.

These believers are like the Galatians who reverted to living by Jewish law. Let's read what Paul wrote to them in Galatians 5:16-18, 22-23:

> This I say then, Walk in the Spirit, and ye shall not fulfil the lust of the flesh. For the flesh lusteth against the Spirit, and the Spirit against the flesh: and these are contrary the one to the other: so that ye cannot do the things that ye would. But if ye be led of the Spirit, ye are not under the law....But the fruit of the Spirit is love, joy, peace, longsuffering, gentleness, goodness, faith, Meekness, temperance: against such there is no law.

According to that scripture, if you're led by your spirit, there won't be any need to impose law on your flesh because your spirit man has been reborn. He's not going to break the law of God—it's written on his

85

heart. (See Hebrews 8:10.) He has the Spirit of God living in there with him teaching him.

I'll tell you something else that's exciting. If you'll develop your spirit man and put him in charge of your body instead of vice versa, eventually you'll be able to train that body to work with your spirit instead of against it. (That is great news to me. I get tired of fighting my flesh!)

Hebrews 5:13-14 says, *"For every one that useth milk is unskilful in the word of righteousness: for he is a babe. But strong meat belongeth to them that are of full age, even those who by reason of use have their senses exercised to discern both good and evil."*

Practice, Practice, Practice!

Let's look at those verses again. How do they say to bring your senses in line? First, by becoming skilful in the word of righteousness; and second, by reason of use, or by practice.

You have to practice walking in the things of the Spirit. Practice walking by faith. Practice walking in love. Practice, practice, practice!

At first, your flesh will rebel against it. It's not been trained that way and it will be contrary for a while. Some people don't realize that; therefore they get discouraged when they stumble around and fall the first few times they try to walk by the Spirit in some area.

They're like a little boy I heard about who used to bat cross-handed. He couldn't get a full swing at the ball because he had his grip reversed. One day his dad said, "Son, don't bat like that. Put your hands the right way so you can swing all the way around."

"I can't hit anything that way!" the boy protested.

"Yes, you can. Come on, I'll show you." The dad helped the boy get his hands right, then backed off and pitched a ball to him. When the boy swung and missed, he threw the bat down in disgust and said, "See there, I told you I couldn't hit anything like that!"

That's the way some Christians are. They decide to walk in love; mess up once and then say, "See there, I knew I couldn't do it!"

Don't be that way. Keep practicing. Pick out some old boy that's nearly impossible to love and start practicing on him. If you strike out the first time at bat, don't worry about it. There's more than three strikes in this game. You just keep swinging until you hit.

Somebody once asked me, "Don't you ever have any failures?" No, I don't, because I don't play nine-inning games. We play until I win. I have a lot of opportunities to fail if I received failure. My shortcomings are many. I've fallen on my face many times. But I don't count that as failure. I just count that as practice. But when I win, praise God, that's for real!

"But Brother Copeland, that's not playing fair." You show me in the Word of God where it says we have to play fair with the devil. I don't play fair with him. I go in with a stacked deck. I go in with the Name of Jesus that's above every name. There's nothing fair about that. But that's okay because the devil is already whipped. We don't have to play fair with him anymore, we just go in and exercise the victory.

No Condemnation Allowed

There's one serious mistake we've made right here that has tripped us up in the past and kept us from playing until we win and it's this: We've let the devil put us under condemnation.

Romans 8:1 says, *"There is therefore now no condemnation to them which are in Christ Jesus, who walk not after the flesh, but after the Spirit."* The condemnation of the carnal mind will weaken the spirit man. Yet we use condemnation on ourselves and each other all the time.

Say, for example, a young man makes Jesus the Lord of his life. He's just gotten up from the altar. He has long hair, dirty feet and a pack of cigarettes he'll probably smoke as soon as he leaves the church. Don't you start condemning him for those things.

That man is walking in the Spirit in all the light he has.

Now, as he hears the Word of God on deliverance one of these days, he'll reach in his pocket and pitch those cigarettes away. He won't need those anymore.

That's what happened to me. I fought cigarettes with everything I had. I threw away more of them than I smoked. I knew I ought not to be smoking those things. Yet I went from smoking a pack and a half a day to three packs a day after I got saved.

Some people would say that was proof I wasn't saved, but they'd be wrong. I was born again. I knew it!

Two and a half months later, I received the Baptism in the Holy Spirit and spoke with other tongues. Still, I was fighting those cigarettes with both hands and feet. Why? My spirit was trying to get me to believe God and quit, but my body was fighting to keep doing what it had been trained to do.

I was torn between the two. Every time I would light a cigarette, it would just tear me up inside. Yet I was walking in all the light I had. I didn't know how to break the power of that thing.

I finally went to a meeting in Houston, Texas, and heard godly men preach under the anointing of God that Jesus was coming back. You know, the Word says when a man puts his hope in the return of Jesus, it will purify him, and that's what it did for me. I walked away from that meeting without any desire for tobacco. Years have come and gone since then and I haven't had any desire for it at all.

My flesh had to get in line once this spirit man (the real me) was fed the food of the Word of God. It had to yield.

What you need to do is develop your own spirit and become skillful in the Word of righteousness in this area. Learn to confess, "There is no condemnation to those who are in Christ Jesus—and that's me. Therefore, there is no condemnation to me, praise God. I'm walking after the dictates of my spirit, not after the dictates of my flesh."

Then turn your ear off to anybody who tries to condemn you.

If you think I'm giving you license to sin, you're wrong. (I've found people don't need it. They sin without a license all the time.) I'm taking for granted you've come to know that sin doesn't work and that you're looking for a way to stop sinning.

With that said, what you need to realize is that you don't need somebody feeding you condemnation because of your flesh. You need somebody feeding you the righteousness of the Word of God so you can take authority over that flesh.

There may be some things in your life that are a little slow coming around. You will have to resist the devil in those areas. But you can stand against him. You can take the Word of God and put him out.

In the meantime, do not allow yourself to be subjected to harassment or condemnation whether it be physical or spiritual. It's dangerous.

Some years ago, there was a nurse who walked into a hospital room where some friends and I were praying for a man. You could tell when she came in that she would have given anything to join in on our prayer. Finally, one of the men turned to her and asked if she knew the Lord Jesus Christ. "Well, I used to know Him," she answered as tears started running down her cheeks. "But I'm beyond salvation now."

"What do you mean you're beyond salvation?" asked my friend. "What in the world did you do?"

Do you know what it was? She cut her hair! Now that may sound ridiculous to you, but to her it was very real. People in her denomination had so condemned her for cutting her hair that she believed with all her heart she was going to hell.

You can see how that kind of condemnation weakens a person's spirit. Satan uses it to get them to a point where they think, *Well, I'm going to hell anyway. I might as well just sin some more.* Of course, that's a lie. The deeper they get into sin, the more condemned they get and the devil just keeps tightening down the noose until it kills them.

Don't let yourself be subjected to that kind of condemnation. Don't believe it. Don't let yourself or anyone else say things like, "I'm so unworthy. I'm so bad. I'm so worthless." That's against the Word of God. If Jesus walked through the door and stood right here for the next 20 years, preaching every minute of every day, He would never call you unworthy. I can prove it to you in Hebrews 2:11. It says *he is not ashamed to call them [us] brethren.*

If Jesus isn't ashamed of you, then you don't have any business being ashamed of yourself!

So stop it and start believing what the Bible says. Believe that you're God's workmanship created in Christ Jesus. Start confessing that. Instead of talking about what a messed-up rascal you are, start agreeing with the Word and calling yourself the righteousness of God in Christ Jesus (2 Corinthians 5:21). Practice seeing yourself that way. Practice seeing yourself operating in the victory. After all, Jesus has already won it for you. So receive that victory by faith.

One time a fellow came up to me and said, "Brother Copeland, I'll tell you what my problem is. It's my flesh."

I said, "Well, overcome it."

"But, you don't understand!"

"No, but Jesus does," I answered. "And He said He's already overcome the world. So go get in the Word, pray, believe God and walk on off from that problem. The power is within you to do it."

Suddenly it hit him what I was saying. He stopped being hung up on the problem and started focusing on the answer.

That's what you need to do. Quit seeing yourself defeated by your flesh and start seeing yourself like the Word says you are— raised up together with Jesus and seated with Him in heavenly places! (See Ephesians 2:6.) Get your perspective on things from that heavenly position with Him.

Meditate in the Word and give your spirit man something to grow on. As 1 Peter 2:2 says, *"desire the sincere milk of the word, that ye may grow thereby."* Then move on to the *"strong meat [of the Word which] belongeth to them that are of full age, even those who by reason of use have their senses exercised to discern both good and evil"* (Hebrews 5:14).

Bring your spirit man into ascendancy over your mind and your body. You'll still have to fight the fight of faith to keep them in line. But if you're walking in the Spirit, you'll win every time. With a healthy Word-controlled, obedient body, you'll be glad you did.

You'll Never Have to Wonder Again

"...He was wounded for our transgressions, he was bruised for our iniquities: the chastise-ment of our peace was upon him; and with his stripes we are healed."

— ISAIAH 53:5

Gloria
Copeland

Have you ever heard a group of people discussing someone else's tragic illness? Inevitably, one of them will shake their head and say, "Doesn't God work in mysterious ways?"

Then another from that same group will start praying, "God, if it's Your will, please heal so-and-so," as if they're not at all certain whether it's God's will or not.

If you've heard that kind of thing very much, you may well be wondering what to believe about the issue of sickness and disease. So let me help set things straight today: Sickness and disease are not the will of God. They never have been and they never will be. They're contrary to His will. How do I know? Because I've checked out the places where God's will is perfectly demonstrated and I found that sickness and disease weren't there.

Take heaven, for example. God's will is carried out there perfectly. Is there sickness in heaven? Of course not!

"But Gloria," you say, "maybe God's will for earth and God's will for heaven are different."

Jesus obviously didn't think so. He taught His disciples to pray for God's will to be done *"in earth, as it is in heaven"* (Matthew 6:10).

If you need more evidence that sickness isn't part of God's will, take a look at the Garden of Eden before the Fall of Man. God created that garden according to His own will. Everything He put there was good— just like in heaven. There was no death, no sorrow, no sickness and disease, no lack of any kind. Health, happiness and prosperity were there in abundance. Why? Because that's what God wanted for man. It was His will then, and it still is now.

The Bible says God never changes (James 1:17). He couldn't change because He was right the first time. He has never changed His will, never changed His direction, never changed His plan for man.

The reason there's sickness and disease on the earth now is not because God's will changed. It's because man (who had been given dominion over the earth) stepped outside of that will through disobedience. Ever since the day that Adam and Eve yielded themselves to Satan in the garden, God's will has not been done on the earth as a whole.

You may be wondering, *If that's the case, won't I have to put up with sickness and disease as long as I live on the earth?*

No, you won't!

Jesus came to earth and gave Himself as a sacrifice for sin in order to buy back for you everything that Adam lost. He came to destroy all the works of the devil—sickness and disease included! Isaiah 53:5 says, *"He was wounded for our transgressions, he was bruised for our iniquities: the chastisement of our peace was upon him; and with his stripes we are healed."*

Once you receive Jesus as Lord of your life, you're made right with God again. All the rights and privileges God originally intended you to have (the right to things like fellowship with God, health and prosperity) are restored.

"If that's true, then why are so many believers still sick?"

Because many have never exercised those rights!

You see, even though Jesus has already defeated the devil and taken away his authority in the earth, He's instructed us to enforce that defeat. The devil has no legal right to kill or steal from the children of God, but he's an outlaw! So he'll do it anyway as long as we'll let him get away with it.

We've got to enforce his defeat by speaking the Word of God in faith. As James 4:7 says, we've got to resist the devil and he will flee from us.

If you don't know how to do that, you'd better find out because as long as you remain passive, Satan will put sickness and disease on you every chance he gets. Ignorance is not bliss when it comes to spiritual things.

I've heard people say, "We did all we knew to do and that person died anyway." In the first place that is rarely ever true. Most of the time people do all that is comfortable to do and that is entirely different. Other times Christians might do all they know, but the problem is that they just don't know enough.

That's the reason God commands us to be diligent in His Word. We need to find out how God operates and how He wants us to operate. The more time we spend in His Word learning about that, the more victorious we're going to be.

This is serious business. Hosea 4:6 says, *"My [God's] people are destroyed for lack of knowledge!"* That's why so many die before their days are fulfilled. Not because it's God's will—but for lack of knowledge. They don't know the Word of God.

Jesus knew the Word of God and the will of God perfectly. He understood that sickness was a work of the devil. So He demonstrated

God's will by setting people free from sickness and disease at every opportunity.

Colossians 1:15 says that Jesus is *"the exact likeness of the unseen God..." (The Amplified Bible)*. That means you can see what God does by watching what Jesus does. And do you know what? Jesus healed everyone who came to Him in faith.

He never refused to heal anyone. He never said, "I'm sorry. I guess you'll have to keep that sickness because God has sent it to you for a purpose."

No! The Bible says:

> **Jesus went forth...moved with compassion...and he healed their sick...And great multitudes came unto him, having with them those that were lame, blind, dumb, maimed, and many others, and cast them down at Jesus' feet; and he healed them: Insomuch that the multitude wondered, when they saw the dumb to speak, the maimed to be whole, the lame to walk, and the blind to see:**

and they glorified the God of Israel (Matthew 14:14, 15:30-31).

Religious tradition says that God gets glory when we bear up nobly under the agony of sickness and disease. But that's not what the Bible says. It says God gets glory when the blind see and the lame walk and the maimed are made whole!

And speaking of religious tradition, have you noticed that religious people always talk about the good old days when God did mighty miracles? They also talk about the great things He's going to do in the future. But when you start talking about now, they get upset. When you say Jesus heals today, they don't want to hear that.

Jesus ran into that situation. In His hometown of Nazareth, people were religious. They believed the Word of God—as long as it pertained to yesterday or tomorrow. But when Jesus told them, *"TODAY is this scripture fulfilled in your ears,"* they got mad. And, the Bible says that as a result, Jesus was able to do no mighty works among them.

You can see that same principle at work in the world today. You can go preach the Word of God to religious folks—you can open the Bible and read it right to them—and they'll get all huffy and tell you that what you just read has passed away. They'll insist that God doesn't do those kinds of things anymore. What's more, they'll be proven right every time because their attitude will keep God from working even one miracle among them, just like it did at Nazareth.

But in Africa where people haven't been taught such religious traditions, when somebody stands up and announces, "I come to you as a messenger from the Most High God," people believe what he has to say. When they hear that Jesus, Lord of lords and King of kings and Son of the Most High God, shed His blood for them, when they hear He's sent His messenger to tell them that He'll deliver them from sin and sickness and death today, they get excited.

They don't sit there and think, *Well now, that's not what my denomination teaches.*

They don't argue with the Word of God. They just believe it and people begin to get healed. People start throwing away their crutches and flinging off their bandages. They don't argue with the man of God. They believe him. That's why people get such dramatic results in countries like Africa. Simple faith is the result because the people just believe what they hear without reservation.

When we learn to hear the Word of God like that, the same thing will happen where you live. God is no respecter of persons. If He'll do that in Africa, He'll do it in Oklahoma City or Chicago or San Francisco. God is the same. It's how we receive the Word that makes the difference.

I want to give you a chance right now to receive God's Word like that. The Bible says, "By His stripes you were healed." Your healing has been bought and paid for by Jesus Christ. It belongs to you.

You may say, "Well, I sure don't feel healed." Listen. This is the Word of the Most High God. You act on it. Demand that sickness and disease leave you in the Name of Jesus. Resist the devil with all you've got, and he can't stay in your mind or on your body.

If you believe this good news I'm telling you, I want you to do something right now. I want you to stand up. Right there, with this book still in your hand, stand on your feet.

Now I want you to say aloud:

"This gospel that I've heard is the power of God toward me. I confess Jesus Christ is Lord over my life—spirit, soul and body. I receive the power of God to make me sound, whole, delivered, saved and healed right now.

"Sickness, disease and pain, I resist you in the Name of Jesus. I enforce the Word of God on you. I won't tolerate you in my life. LEAVE MY PRESENCE. Jesus has already borne my sickness, my weakness and pain, and I am free.

"Sickness shall no longer lord it over me. Sin shall no longer lord it over me. Fear shall no longer lord it over me. I have been redeemed. I proclaim my freedom in Jesus' Name."

Now, don't ever look back. God's will is exactly the same now as it was in the Garden of Eden and in the life of Jesus. God's will is for you to be free. Rejoice. Believe the message. You'll never have to wonder again.

God's Medicine!

Chapter 8

"Death and life are in the power of the tongue: and they that love it shall eat the fruit thereof."
— PROVERBS 18:21

Charles Capps

Medical science tells us there are many incurable diseases, such as some forms of cancer, arthritis, heart disease and AIDS, just to name a few. Even though there are no known medical cures for these diseases, God's Word is a supernatural cure and offers supernatural hope to all who are afflicted.

There is probably no other subject as important to healing and health than the principle of calling things that are not. This one principle could be the key to your being a partaker of God's provisions concerning your healing.

Calling things that are not is the principle by which Abraham became fully persuaded that God would do what He had promised. Paul said that Abraham believed

God, *"who quickeneth the dead, and calleth those things which be not as though they were"* (Romans 4:17).

Here Paul is referring to Genesis 17. God called Abram the father of nations *before* he had the promised child, and He taught Abram to do the same.

God changed Abram's name to *Abraham*, which meant "father of nations, or multitude." This was the means He used to convince Abraham to call for what he did not yet have in reality. God had established it by promise, but Abram had to call it into reality by mixing faith with God's Word.

Every time he said, "I am Abraham," he was calling things that were not yet manifest. Abraham did not deny that he was old. He didn't go around saying, "I'm not old," because he was old. But he said, "I am Abraham," (Father of Nations). This was God's method of helping him change his image, and it caused him to be fully persuaded.

Just as Abraham, you also must call those things which are not yet seen in the natural, if you are to live in the reality of God's promise.

For God uses unseen spiritual forces to overcome natural things. First Corinthians 1:27-28 says, *"God hath chosen...things which are not, to bring to nought things that are."*

Your part is to speak what is true according to God's Word.

David said, *"I believed, therefore have I spoken..."* (Psalm 116:10). Quoting David, Paul wrote, *"We having the same spirit of faith, according as it is written, I believed, and therefore have I spoken; we also believe, and therefore speak"* (2 Corinthians 4:13).

When it comes to divine healing, this is a vital principle. For God's Word is life, health, and medicine to all your flesh.

Psalm 107:20 tells us that God *"sent his word, and healed them, and delivered them from their destructions."* (Notice that God did not send His Word to heal, but He sent His *Word and healed*.)

The truth is that by Jesus' stripes *"ye were healed"* (1 Peter 2:24). Your healing is a complete work as far as God's Word is concerned. Yet we must be fully persuaded of it and call it into manifestation.

Healing Is in Your Mouth

One way to administer God's medicine to your body is to keep God's Word in your mouth. For Paul said, "The Word is nigh you even in your mouth and then in your heart." But, instead of calling things that are not, most people make the mistake of calling things the way they are.

I read an article many years ago about a lady who had a fever continually for several months. Doctors couldn't find anything wrong physically.

They questioned her thoroughly and discovered that when she got upset about anything, she would always say, "That just burns me up." She used that phrase several times a day. The doctors were not sure if it had anything to do with her condition or not, but they asked her not to use the phrase anymore.

Within weeks, her body temperature was normal.

Now let me ask you, how many times have you said, "Every time I eat that, it makes me sick...My back is just killing me... Those kids make me so nervous...I'm trying to take the flu...."? Your own words are giving instructions to your body. Eventually your immune system will respond to your instructions and you will have what you have been saying.

God's method is to call for positive things, even though they are not yet a reality in your body. Call them until they are manifested. Exercise your God-given authority over your body.

Apply Spiritual Medicine

To exercise your authority over your body, God's Word must be allowed to become part of you. This process is called receiving the engrafted Word.

Just as you would take medicine into your physical body to aid healing by physical means, so you must receive God's Word concerning healing into your spirit for supernatural healing. Just as medical science aids healing through physical means by administering medicine into the physical body, God's medicine provides divine healing by administering the promises of

His Word through the human spirit. God's Word will heal your body, but it does it through spiritual means.

Although it is a spiritual cure, God's Word is like any other medicine—in that it must be applied on a regular basis. You must apply God's Word to your individual circumstance or situation by the confession of your mouth. No one else can do it for you. James admonished us to *"receive with meekness the engrafted word, which is able to save your souls"* (James 1:21).

God's Word becomes engrafted into your heart as you speak it. It is first in your mouth, then in the heart...this is God's order.

"The righteousness which is of faith... says...The word is nigh thee, even in thy mouth, and in thy heart..." (Romans 10:6-8). Nothing builds up your faith more than declaring with your own voice what God has said about you in His Word.

When you declare God's promises concerning your healing, you are establishing God's truth even before it is reality in your body. This is not denying that sickness exists. It is denying sickness the right to exist in your body. It is taking your rightful position as one who has been redeemed from the curse of the law and delivered from the authority of darkness (Galatians 3:13; Colossians 1:13).

Some people who have misunderstood this principle try to deny what exists. But there is no power in denying what exists. The power is in calling for healing and health, and you do that by mixing your faith with God's Word.

If you are sick, you don't deny that you are sick. On the other hand, you don't want to always be confessing your sickness. Denying sickness will not make you well, yet confessing sickness establishes you in your present circumstance and gives you a mind-set of fear.

Make a decision to mix your faith with God's Word and call for God's promises to be manifest in your body. The mixing of your faith with God's Word will cause you to be fully persuaded. When you become fully persuaded, healing is the result.

Do you want your flesh to reflect the life of God's Word? Let the Word become so infused into your spirit that it becomes a part of you. Not only will His Word become your thought and affirmation...but it will be you. When God's Word concerning healing takes root in your flesh, it becomes greater than pain, greater than disease, and God's Word through your words is made flesh!

Seeing Yourself Whole

When the Word of God is allowed to be engrafted into you, it creates in you an image of what is already reality in the spirit realm. When you speak that Word from your heart, then faith gives substance to the promises of God. Those images become stronger every time you speak your faith.

A healing image is created in you by God's Word and your continual affirmation and agreement with what God has said. That image is perfected by the Word of God until you begin to see yourself well. The Word engrafted into you is infusing its life into you (John 6:63; Romans 8:11).

This was demonstrated by the woman with the issue of blood, who followed Jesus saying, *"If I may touch but his clothes, I shall be whole"* (Mark 5:28). The verb tense is made more clear in *The Amplified Bible,* which says, *"For she kept saying, If I only touch His garments, I shall be restored to health."*

This woman hoped to be healed as she pressed through the crowd. She continued to speak until she saw herself well. Her hope was that she would be healed, although she didn't feel or look healed. But she began filling her hope with faith-filled words: "I shall be restored to health...I shall be restored to health...I shall be...I shall be...."

I'm sure her head demanded, *When? You don't look any better.* So she answered human reasoning by filling her hope with a faith image: *When I touch His garments.*

Those words penetrated her spirit and she began to see herself well. Images of despair and defeat gave way to faith-filled words. When she touched Jesus' garments, her touch of faith made a demand on the covenant of God and on the healing anointing that was upon Jesus. As faith gave substance to her hope, healing was manifested in her body.

Hope is a goal setter, but it lacks substance until it is filled with faith. Faith gave substance to her hope, laid claim to what was hers according to the promises of His covenant, and brought manifestation of her healing. *"Daughter, thy faith hath made thee whole."* Jesus told her (verse 34). *"Whosoever shall say...he shall have..."* (Mark 11:23). These are Bible principles of believing and calling for things that are not yet manifest.

The Language of Health

The words you speak are vital to your health and well-being. I believe there are some diseases that will never be cured unless people learn to speak the language of health that the body understands. That language of health is the engrafting of God's Word into you by giving voice to His Word with your own mouth.

Your words become either a curse or a blessing to you. I am convinced from my study of the Word of God that your own words can change your immune system for better or worse. (See James 3:2-7.)

Proverbs 18:21 tells us that *"Death and life are in the power of the tongue: and they that love it shall eat the fruit thereof."* In a recent study, men and women 65 and older were asked to rate their health as excellent, good, fair or poor.

The study showed that those who rated their health as poor were four to five times more likely to die within four years as those who rated themselves as excellent. This was true even when examinations showed the respondents to be in comparable health.

People who have an image of themselves being in poor health will talk about poor health. Even though they may be in good health, they seem to live out the reality of the image they have of themselves even unto death.

On the other hand, I believe that people who continually affirm the Word in faith will build into their immune systems a supernatural anointing that is capable of eliminating sickness and disease in a natural manner.

By being taught properly and by practicing your faith, you can grow to the point where it will be a common thing for you to receive healing through the Word of God. Yet, this doesn't happen overnight. Use some common sense and don't do foolish things through spiritual pride and call it faith.

It takes time to develop faith to operate in these principles, so don't let anyone put you under condemnation for going to doctors or having an operation. You must operate on your level of faith, but don't stay on that level forever. Continue in God's Word until you develop faith in the healing power of God's Word.

Confess the promises of God's Word concerning your health and healing daily. Confess the Word audibly over your body two or three times a day. Confess it with authority. Confessing God's Word is a way you can fellowship with the Lord and increase your faith at the same time.

Take God's Word on a regular basis, just as you would take any other medicine. Practice God's medicine; it is life to you and health to your flesh.

Chapter 9

Four Steps to Lasting Results

"For whatsoever is born of God overcometh the world: and this is the victory that overcometh the world, even our faith. Who is he that overcometh the world, but he that believeth that Jesus is the Son of God?"

— 1 John 5:4-5

Marty Copeland

I've got good news! Jesus wants you to be free from every kind of bondage—whether it be overeating, cigarette smoking, alcohol abuse or fear that you'll gain back the weight you've lost. But before you start a regular exercise plan and change your habits, be sure to put these four steps to work for you so your results will last.

1. Make Jesus Your Lord (1 John 5:1-4)

Making Jesus Lord over everything in your life—from your spirit to your physical body—will be the best decision you've ever made. It's also a very necessary decision in order to involve God's anointing in your freedom. Isaiah 10:27 says God's anointing is His burden-removing, yoke-destroying power...and it's just what you need to stop the power of sin and death once and for all.

2. Put Your Hope and Faith in God
(2 Corinthians 10:4-5)

Too many times we put our hope in carnal weapons—diets, pills, certain kinds of exercise—and then, by faith, we believe that those things are going to win our warfare. But when you put your hope and faith in carnal things, there's no substance... you're deceived into fighting a spiritual warfare in the arena of the flesh. So put your hope and faith in God. It's the only sure way to lasting victory.

3. Realize the Past Doesn't Matter
(2 Corinthians 5:17)

Once you were born again, all things became new. You were reborn with right-standing before God, and you received all the ability it takes to walk in victory all the days of your life. It doesn't matter how many times you've failed, put your hope in

a weight-loss product or anything else...
because now you can do all things through
the Anointed One and His Anointing.

4. Walk in the Spirit (Galatians 5:16)

When you walk in the Spirit, you won't
fulfill the lust of the flesh. Instead, you'll
begin to develop the fruit of the Spirit as
you fill yourself with God's Word and
discover who you are in Christ. And it's the
fruit of the Spirit—patience, faithfulness
and self-control—that gives you the power
to overcome.

So get your hope off diets, "fast fixes"
and carnal weapons today...and put your
hope in God. Because when you put your
hope and faith in Him, you'll release the
power of His yoke-destroying anointing
to produce burden-removing results that
will last!

Entering God's Rest— What a Way to Live!

Chapter 10

"Come unto me, all ye that labour and are heavy laden, and I will give you rest."
— MATTHEW 11:28

Kenneth Copeland

These days a great many Christians— good, God-loving folks—are extremely weary. They shouldn't be. But they are.

I'm not criticizing them, because there have been times in the past when I felt like the most tired of the bunch. I was once so tired, I asked God to let me go on to heaven so I could get some rest.

Of course, He didn't pay any attention to that request. What He did instead was show me how to be free from that fatigue. He revealed to me through His Word that I didn't have to put off resting until I got to heaven. I could—and should—be resting here and now.

That's right. Hebrews 4:3 says, *"we which have believed do enter into rest."* It doesn't say we will enter rest someday. It says we do enter it today.

Granted, the whole idea of resting is strange to most of the Body of Christ. Religion has so robbed us of the rest of God that most of us haven't even known that rest was available...much less how to enter into it.

But, the fact is, God's rest is ours if we'll do what it takes to enter it. So if you've been tired—tired of struggling and striving and worrying—and you'd like to kick back and enjoy your life in God for a change, pay attention here. You're about to learn how to do it.

A Day in the Life of Jesus

Someone might say, "Well now, Brother Copeland, you wouldn't be so quick to tell me I could rest if you knew my schedule. The demands of my life and ministry are overwhelming. The devil is hounding me from every side and my circumstances are really rough. There's no way anyone could rest in the middle of all this."

Jesus could. We know He could because when we read the New Testament, we see times when He faced those same situations. Matthew 8 gives us a glimpse of one of those times. Let's read it and see what we can learn:

> And when Jesus was come into Peter's house, he saw his wife's mother laid, and sick of a fever. And he touched her hand, and the fever left her: and she arose, and ministered unto them. When the even was come, they brought unto him many that were possessed with devils: and he cast out the spirits with his word, and healed all that were sick: That it might be fulfilled which was spoken by Esaias the prophet, saying, Himself took our infirmities, and bare our sicknesses.
>
> Now when Jesus saw great multitudes about him, he gave commandment to depart unto the other side.... And when he was entered into a ship,

his disciples followed him. And, behold, there arose a great tempest in the sea, insomuch that the ship was covered with the waves: but he was asleep. And his disciples came to him, and awoke him, saying, Lord, save us: we perish. And he saith unto them, Why are ye fearful, O ye of little faith? Then he arose, and rebuked the winds and the sea; and there was a great calm. But the men marvelled, saying, What manner of man is this, that even the winds and the sea obey him! (verses 14-18, 23-27).

Actually, to see the complete picture of this particular day in Jesus' life, you need to start in Matthew 5 because that day didn't start with the healing of Peter's mother-in-law. It started with Jesus going up onto the mountain and preaching one of the most extensive messages recorded in the New Testament. I'm sure that meeting took up much of the day.

When he was finished, Jesus came down and headed for Peter's house, no doubt so He could rest and eat supper. But He was delayed because on the way, He was approached by a man with leprosy and by a Roman centurion whose sick servant needed healing. Jesus ministered to both those situations, then headed on to the house.

When He got there, He found Peter's mother-in-law was sick. So He ministered to her. She got out of bed healed, and prepared their evening meal. But Jesus' ministry that day still wasn't finished.

When evening came, multitudes came to the door. Many of them were sick. Others were demon possessed. Don't you know that was a welcome sight after such a full day?

But Jesus didn't fall on His face and cry and kick the dirt. He didn't throw a fit and say, "Oh God, I'm so exhausted. I hope I have enough anointing left to heal all these people. I've already been preaching and healing all day long. These people just expect too much of me!"

No, He didn't say any of those things. He just went outside and did the work His Father had given Him to do. He healed the sick and cast out devils.

When He finished, He didn't get to climb into a soft, warm bed, either. He got into a boat and a storm hit. Circumstances were so bad, His disciples were sure they would all die. But what was He doing? He was sleeping.

There in that boat, with the wind howling around Him and the waves slapping over the side, soaking Him with water, He was at rest. Think about that. He wasn't in a cabin cruiser. He was out there exposed to the elements, but they didn't bother Him one bit.

Believe and Obey

How did Jesus enjoy that kind of rest in the midst of those kinds of situations? He did it by faith.

Jesus was full of faith and had entered into the rest of His Father. That was why He could lay down in the back of the boat and go to sleep. The disciples could have enjoyed that same kind of rest if they'd used that same kind of faith.

"Oh, Brother Copeland, surely you don't think the disciples could have done what Jesus did!"

Why not? They had been given a faith command by the Son of the living God. He had told them to go to the other side of that lake. So they had the power and authority to do it. That must be true. Otherwise, Jesus didn't have any right to get on to them for being afraid.

The only obstacle that stood between the disciples and the rest of God was their "little faith." Jesus had big faith, so He had big rest. They had little faith, so they had little rest.

Remember that: Big faith—big rest. Little faith—little rest.

It was big faith that enabled Jesus to teach and minister to the multitudes from morning till night—and do it in the rest of God. It was faith that kept Him from being overwhelmed with the needs of the people.

It was Jesus' faith in His Heavenly Father that kept Him at rest—regardless of the circumstances. Jesus, even though He is

131

the sinless, spotless Son of God, didn't carry out His ministry trusting in His own divine abilities. On the contrary, the Bible says He laid aside the privileges of deity before He came to the earth. So He ministered not as God, but as a man in covenant with God.

Jesus wasn't trusting in Himself. In fact, He said, "I do nothing of Myself. It's the Father in Me that does the works."

Jesus' faith was in the Word of God and in the anointing of God within and upon Him. He knew that anointing would supply the power to bring God's Word to pass. So He had nothing to worry about!

He didn't have to heal anyone. All He had to do was what God said to do, and go where He said to go...and God Himself would take care of the rest. God was the One Who did the healing. God was the One Who stopped the waves. All Jesus had to do was believe and obey.

Notice, I said He obeyed. Sometimes we take for granted Jesus' unquestioning obedience to God. We assume it was easier for Him to obey than it is for us. But think about it for a moment.

Jesus was physically tired that evening. I'm sure He would have enjoyed spending the night at Peter's dry, comfortable house. It would have been reasonable for Him to say, "I'm having a good meeting here. The crowds are good. People are getting healed and delivered. I believe I'll just stay here and keep this meeting going for a few days."

But Jesus didn't do what was comfortable. He didn't do what was reasonable. He did what the Spirit of God told Him to do. So He left a good meeting and a good bed, crossed the lake in bad weather in the middle of the night, and went to face two demon-possessed people and a whole city of pig-loving unbelievers (see Matthew 8:28-34).

Jesus knew that no matter what natural evidence there might be to the contrary, as long as He obeyed God in faith, He didn't have to concern Himself with the outcome of any situation. He knew God had it well in hand, and He could enjoy complete rest.

What Do You Have to Worry About?

The same thing is true for us as believers. If we'll just believe the Word of God and obey Him, we can have the sweetest, most restful life imaginable, and kick the stuffing out of the devil while we're at it!

I realize that's hard for some Christians to swallow. They've been so brainwashed with religious tradition over the years that real spiritual truth goes down hard. They can't imagine how they could ever live like Jesus did. After all, He was Jesus! They're unworthy worms! They're just old sinners saved by grace.

That's what religion has told them. But that's not what the Bible tells us. It says we're united with Jesus. We are one Body with Him. As Hebrews 2:11 says, *"...both he that sanctifieth and they who are sanctified are all of one: for which cause he is not ashamed to call them brethren."*

You can live in Jesus' own rest because, if you've made Him Lord of your life, you're one with Him. The New Testament says again and again, you are in Him. That means you are everything to God that Jesus is. You have His Name. You're washed in His blood. You're in His house.

God loves you every bit as much as He loves Jesus (John 17:23). It seems almost unthinkable, but it's true. And if God loves us just like He loves Jesus, if He's given us His Word, and His anointing, what could we possibly have to worry about?

Nothing, man! Absolutely nothing!

Since we're one with Jesus, we ought to be acting just like Jesus acts. We ought to be living just like He lives. Do you think He's running around heaven, wringing His hands with worry? Do you think He's looking at circumstances down here on earth saying, "Oh, no. It's looking really bad on earth. I'm not sure God will be able to pull off His plan now. I'm not sure His plan is going to turn out the way He said."

Hardly!

The Bible says God sits in the heavens and laughs at His enemies. He's not worried, He's laughing—and Jesus is right beside

Him. Hebrews 10:12-13 shows us exactly what He is doing: *"But this man [Jesus], after he had offered one sacrifice for sins for ever, sat down on the right hand of God; From henceforth expecting till his enemies be made his footstool."*

Jesus is sitting down, expecting! He is at rest, expecting everything to turn out exactly as God has said.

That's exactly what we need to be doing. God has *"raised us up together, and made us sit together in heavenly places in Christ Jesus"* (Ephesians 2:6). So we don't have any more business wringing our hands than Jesus Himself does! We should be at rest, expecting the devil and all his works to be put under our feet!

Labor to Enter the Rest

I realize that sounds easier said than done. But it can be done if we will just do it! Hebrews 4:9-11 tells us how: *"There remaineth therefore a rest to the people of God. For he that is entered into his rest, he also hath ceased from his own works, as*

God did from his [on the seventh day of creation]. Let us labour therefore to enter into that rest, lest any man fall after the same example of unbelief."

We have to labor to enter the rest. We have to stop struggling and striving to handle things in our own human wisdom and strength. We have to stop trying to wrestle our circumstances to the ground. Instead, we must labor spiritually and do what it takes to walk in faith.

We must read and meditate on the Word, and fellowship with the Lord over it—then cast down every thought contrary to His Word. We must stay in the Word and on our knees until faith rises in our hearts. We must keep at it until we can look the devil right in the face and laugh with joy because we know the battle has already been won! When we do that, we'll enter into God's rest.

You may be thinking, *Surely he's not serious! My bank account is completely empty and I have a stack of unpaid bills a foot high!...I'm dying and the doctor says there's nothing medicine can do for me!...*

My children are on drugs!...How could I ever laugh with joy in this condition?

By looking to Jesus. He's the author and the finisher of our faith. He's our High Priest. He's the One with Whom we're united. Hebrews 2:17-18 says, *"Wherefore in all things it behoved him to be made like unto his brethren [once more, Jesus and us together], that he might be a merciful and faithful high priest in things pertaining to God, to make reconciliation for the sins of the people. For in that he himself hath suffered being tempted, he is able to succour them that are tempted."*

You may think you're facing the most tremendous problems anyone ever faced. You may think you're under such severe pressure it would be impossible for you to rest in the midst of it. You may think there's no one who can understand, no one who can help you through it.

But Jesus can.

He knows what real pressure is. He has been there, my friend. You and I can't even imagine the kind of pressure Jesus faced.

Consider it for a moment. If we sin, we repent and get cleansed of it. If Jesus had sinned, the whole world would have gone to hell. That's pressure!

He dealt with that pressure in the Garden of Gethsemane. He labored there in prayer and in fellowship with God until He entered God's rest. He stayed there until He could say, *"Thy will be done."* Then He got up and walked out of there for the joy that was set before Him. He went straight to the Cross, through hell, was resurrected and sat down at God's right hand!

"Oh, but that was Jesus!"

That's right. That was Jesus. Your blood Brother. The One Who has declared you sinless, free and just like Him in the presence of Almighty God. The One Who has given you His Spirit. The One Who has given you His Name. The One Who has given you His Word. The One Who has given you His anointing.

So enter His rest! Roll the care of that problem over on Him and expect the victory.

I know it can be done because I've done it. I had to do it years ago when our television bills ran away with us and we found ourselves several million dollars behind. For a good, long time, I took the care of that deficit myself. I worried over it. I tried to figure out how to fix it. I thought about selling the ministry property to pay it.

Then something interesting happened. I received our year-end report and found out we'd had the most productive year in ministry we'd ever had. We only had one major problem—and that was in the area I'd been trying to handle myself.

The Lord said to me, *See there, the area you hung onto is the one that's messed up.*

Immediately, Gloria and I saw what we had to do. We had to take authority over that situation and completely roll the care of it over on the Lord. We had to set our minds and hearts on God's Word and completely get into His rest.

I did it too...for about 30 seconds. Then I started thinking about it again. I was in such a habit of thinking about that deficit, it would slip back into my mind before I even realized it.

So every time it did, I said out loud, "No, that's not my thought. I refuse to think it. Get out of my mind. I bring my thoughts under obedience to the anointing of Jesus. I've rolled the care of this thing over on God and I'm not going to touch it." I did that time after time, day after day. I labored to enter God's rest.

The first week I had to speak out loud to those thoughts of care every few minutes—sometimes every few seconds. By the end of the second week, it was a few times a day.

By the end of the third week, I couldn't have cared less about that deficit. My thoughts had been brought into captivity in obedience to Christ. It wasn't my problem anymore. It was God's and I knew He could handle it.

Sure enough, He did. In six months the deficit was completely paid. What's more, for the first time in the history of this ministry, we were able to start paying our television bills in one payment each month instead of paying them a little at a time throughout the month. And we've been paying that way ever since.

Hallelujah, what a wonderful, powerful, victorious way to live!

Do you want to live that way? You can!

Receive Jesus' anointing in Hebrews 3:1, as your High Priest. Keep your confession right. Keep your faith right. Go boldly before the throne of grace and receive mercy and grace to help in your time of need.

Then rest with Jesus. Sit down with Him, prop your feet up on the devil's head and expect the victory.

God Himself has already guaranteed— it's yours!

A Carefree Life?

Chapter 11

"Humble yourselves therefore under the mighty hand of God, that he may exalt you in due time: Casting all your care upon him; for he careth for you."
— 1 PETER 5:6-7

Kenneth Copeland

Sitting in your living room. A fire roaring in the fireplace. Bills piled to the ceiling. Children running throughout the house. More laundry to do. Plans to make. Details to handle...

Can you really have a peaceful life with all those pressures bearing down on you?

Yes, you can—and you don't have to leave the country to do it. No matter how intense or how trivial the problems are that you're facing right now, you can live the most peaceful, carefree life you've ever lived—and you can start today.

How?

Look at 1 Peter 5:6-7 and I'll show you. It says, *"Humble yourselves therefore under the mighty hand of God, that he may exalt you in due time: Casting all your care upon him; for he careth for you."*

As a believer, you're probably familiar with that scripture. But have you ever taken it seriously enough to put it into action? There's a good chance you haven't because you haven't understood just how dangerous those cares you're carrying around actually are.

You probably haven't realized that they are a deadly part of the devil's strategy against you.

That's right. Worry is one of the chief weapons of his warfare. If he can get you to worry about them, he can use the financial and family pressures and scheduling problems that are just a "normal" part of everyday life to weigh you down, drain your spiritual strength, and drag you into more trouble than you care to think about.

You see, worry produces a deadly force—the force of fear. It is what Satan uses to govern his kingdom. He uses it to kill, steal and destroy. It's a killer force.

That's why all through the Bible the Holy Spirit commands, "FEAR NOT!" He's not just giving friendly advice. He's giving us an order from our Commander in Chief, an order that will keep us from falling prey to the enemy's attack.

Medical science tells us that approximately 80 percent of the people hospitalized in the United States are there with ailments caused by worry and tension. Yet a great many believers worry without even thinking about it.

They'll worry about finding the time to get their hair cut. They'll worry about getting the right present for Grandma's birthday. They'll stew over this and that and then go to church and not even realize they've been sinning all week long!

"Sinning, Brother Copeland?"

Yes! For the born-again, Spirit-filled believer who owns a Bible—worrying is a sin.

I've had people say to me, "Brother Copeland, pray for me that I'll be able to bear these burdens." Well, I won't do it. Jesus said if you're burdened and heavy laden, to come to Him and He'd give you rest. He didn't say, "Pray and I'll give you the strength to bear your burdens." He said, "I'll give you REST!"

Let's get something straight right now. A mind that is burdened down with worry is not a godly mind. You may be born again and baptized in the Holy Spirit, but if your mind is controlled by worry it is not controlled by the Holy Spirit of God.

I don't care how major or minor your problem is, Philippians 4:6 says to be anxious about nothing, but in everything pray and give thanks and make your requests known to God. It doesn't say, "Worry about it for four or five days." It says, "Pray and give thanks."

That means if you're going to obey God, you must make a decision to quit worrying. You must realize that it's part of Satan's strategy.

"But what should I do with my cares," you say, "if I'm not going to worry about them anymore?"

You use the force of faith and do just what Jesus did when the devil came at Him.

Jesus said, *"The prince of this world cometh, and hath nothing in me"* (John 14:30). The devil never could get any of his junk into Jesus. He threw at Him everything he could throw, but Jesus wouldn't let it in.

He'd just say, "No, I don't live by that. I live by the Word, thank you." He wouldn't receive anything the devil said. He just trusted God and said, *"It is written...."*

When the devil attacked Jesus with worry, He didn't give in to it. He fought back with His double-edged sword. He clobbered the devil with the Spirit-power of the Word.

You see, the only way you can truly cast your care on God is by believing what He's already said about that care. The only way you can be free when it comes to finances is by believing that God has met all your needs according to His riches in glory by Christ Jesus (Philippians 4:19). The only way you can cast the care of sickness over on God is by believing that by His stripes you were healed (1 Peter 2:24).

That's why, when the devil wants to destroy you, he'll send a demon spirit to exalt himself against the Word of God.

If you're sick, he'll begin to tell you, "You're not healed. You know healing is not for today. Even if it were, it wouldn't work for you. It might for someone else, but not you."

When he starts to tell you that kind of thing, don't buy into it! Don't start worrying around about it and thinking, *Oh my, I'm afraid I'm not going to get healed. I sure don't feel healed. Why, I'm probably just going to get worse and worse....*

Don't do that! Do as Paul said in 2 Corinthians 10:5: *"Casting down imaginations, and every high thing that exalteth itself against the knowledge of God, and bringing into captivity every thought...."* Hit the devil with the Word, and cast the care of the situation over on God.

If you're thinking, *Yes, that sounds like a good thing to do, but I'm not Jesus! I'm just little old me,* remember that Jesus said He wasn't the One responsible for His success.

He was using the Word of God. He said, *"The Father that dwelleth in me, he doeth the works"* (John 14:10).

Remember that. It's the Word that does the work, not the one holding onto it. It'll work for anyone who will put it to work. It will work for you just like it worked for Jesus. Just put it out there, and then get in behind it and hide. Let the Word fight its own fight.

When I first learned how to do that, I was down in South Texas preaching at a meeting that no one was coming to. I'm telling you, people were staying away from that meeting by the thousands. And after a service or two with just the pastor and me and one or two others there, I was starting to sweat it. But the Lord said, *Cast that care on Me,* so I did.

I started walking around grinning and whistling. I told the devil, "I'm not going to frown or have one worried thought. I came here to preach and that's what I'm going to do. It's God's business whether anyone shows up or not. I could care less!"

I went around so happy I felt downright foolish. The devil said, "What's the matter with you? Don't you even have sense enough to worry over something like this?" News got back to me that some of the people were saying, "I guess he's too dumb to worry. I think it's because he's never been to seminary. He can't tell a landslide from a flop."

But I told the Lord, "I have my care rolled over on You, and if nobody shows up but that one dear old woman, she's going to be the most preached-up old woman in the state of Texas because I'm going to preach just the same as if there was a crowd."

I didn't realize then what was happening, but that carefreeness put me in a noncompromising position with the devil. He couldn't get to me anymore. He couldn't pressure me and get me to compromise because I didn't care! I'd given all my care to God!

Once, when I was preaching in Louisiana, it was the last night of the meeting and the budget hadn't been met. We were $900 short. During those early days, $900 might as well have been $9 million.

The devil was jumping on me so bad I couldn't afford to let my mind run loose five seconds. So I went outside and started walking up and down the motel patio, praising the Lord out loud. I'd found that my tongue controlled my mind.

By the way, if you haven't discovered that, let me demonstrate it really quickly. Start counting silently from one to 10. Now, while you're still counting, say your name out loud. See what I mean? Your head had to stop counting and see what your mouth had to say, didn't it? Use that the next time your mind starts to worry about something. Make it stop by speaking the promises of God out loud.

Anyway, I was walking back and forth out there praying out loud, confessing the Word and praising God. Whenever I'd stop, the devil would say, "You ain't going to get it."

Then I'd say, "As far as I'm concerned I already have it. I prayed and cast that care over on God, and He pays His bills!"

I just kept it up and kept it up, holding the devil over in the arena of faith, rather than letting him pull me over in that arena of worry.

Suddenly a man pulled up into the motel driveway. He honked his horn and stuck his head out the window. "Brother Copeland, I'm so glad I caught you. I had to get by here to see you because I won't get to the meeting until late tonight and I was afraid I might miss the offering."

He held out a check and said, "I wanted to make sure you got this." Then he turned around and drove off. The check was for $500. That night we went over the budget.

You see, God will handle it for you if you cast those cares on Him. Not only that, but He also says He'll exalt you. Exalt you above what? Above the devil and all his crowd. Above every problem he tries to use against you.

That's God's plan for your victory. It doesn't make Him any difference if it's December or the Fourth of July. It doesn't matter if the dog needs a bath, *again,* and everyone on your son's soccer team is coming to your house for dinner. The Bible says, *"...delight thyself in the Lord; and I will cause thee to ride upon the high places of the earth..."* (Isaiah 58:14).

God is an exalter. He wants to lift you above that anxiety and care the devil uses to pull you down. You can understand now why the psalmist says, *"He maketh my feet like hinds' feet..."* (Psalm 18:33). A deer's feet touch the ground every once in a while, but most of the time, they're in the air!

Are you ready to be free of care? If you are, just lift your hands where you're sitting and make this confession of faith: "I'm a believer. I'm not a doubter. The Word works in me; and at this moment, I humble myself under the mighty hand of God. I cast the care of _____ (name it out loud) over on Him. From this moment forward, I refuse to worry. Instead, I will pray. I will use my faith, and He'll exalt me over the problem and over the devil. For I belong to Jesus. He's made me to sit with Him in heavenly places. I've put on the whole armor of God. From this very moment, with Jesus as my helper, I'm carefree. He has my cares. He'll work them out. He'll do it. He'll finish the work."

Shout, "Thank God I don't have a care!"

Now, go ahead and have a truly peaceful life, you carefree thing you!

Prayer for Salvation and Baptism in the Holy Spirit

Heavenly Father, I come to You in the Name of Jesus. Your Word says, *"Whosoever shall call on the name of the Lord shall be saved"* (Acts 2:21). I am calling on You. I pray and ask Jesus to come into my heart and be Lord over my life according to Romans 10:9. *"If thou shalt confess with thy mouth the Lord Jesus, and shalt believe in thine heart that God hath raised him from the dead, thou shalt be saved."* I do that now. I confess that Jesus is Lord, and I believe in my heart that God raised Him from the dead.

I am now reborn! I am a Christian—a child of Almighty God! I am saved! You also said in Your Word, *"If ye then, being evil, know how to give good gifts unto your children: HOW MUCH MORE shall your heavenly Father give the Holy Spirit to them that ask him?"* (Luke 11:13). I'm also asking You to fill me with the Holy Spirit. Holy Spirit, rise up within me as I praise God. I fully expect to speak with other tongues as You give me the utterance (Acts 2:4).

Begin to praise God for filling you with the Holy Spirit. Speak those words and syllables you receive—not in your own language, but the language given to you by the Holy Spirit. You have to use your own voice. God will not force you to speak. Worship and praise Him in your heavenly language—in other tongues.

Continue with the blessing God has given you and pray in tongues each day.

You are a born-again, Spirit-filled believer. You'll never be the same!

Find a good Word of God preaching church, and become a part of a church family who will love and care for you as you love and care for them.

We need to be hooked up to each other. It increases our strength in God. It's God's plan for us.

Books Available From Kenneth Copeland Publications

by Kenneth Copeland
* A Ceremony of Marriage
  A Matter of Choice
  Covenant of Blood
  Faith and Patience—The Power Twins
* Freedom From Fear
  Giving and Receiving
  Honor—Walking in Honesty, Truth and Integrity
  How to Conquer Strife
  How to Discipline Your Flesh
  How to Receive Communion
  Living at the End of Time—A Time of Supernatural
      Increase
  Love Never Fails
  Managing God's Mutual Funds
* Now Are We in Christ Jesus
* Our Covenant With God
* Prayer—Your Foundation for Success
  Prosperity: The Choice Is Yours
  Rumors of War
* Sensitivity of Heart
  Six Steps to Excellence in Ministry
  Sorrow Not! Winning Over Grief and Sorrow
* The Decision Is Yours
* The Force of Faith
* The Force of Righteousness
  The Image of God in You
  The Laws of Prosperity
* The Mercy of God
  The Miraculous Realm of God's Love
  The Outpouring of the Spirit—The Result of Prayer
* The Power of the Tongue
  The Power to Be Forever Free

From Faith to Faith—A Daily Guide to Victory
Over the Edge—Youth Devotional
Pursuit of His Presence—Daily Devotional

Other Books Published by KCP
* Heirs Together by Mac Hammond
Winning the World by Mac Hammond

The First 30 Years—A Journey of Faith
    The story of the lives of Kenneth and
        Gloria Copeland.
Real People. Real Needs. Real Victories.
    A book of testimonies to encourage your faith.

John G. Lake—His Life, His Sermons, His Boldness
    of Faith
The Holiest of All by Andrew Murray
The New Testament in Modern Speech by
    Richard Francis Weymouth

Products Designed by KCP and Heirborne™ for
    Today's Children and Youth

Baby Praise Board Book
Noah's Ark Coloring Book
The *Shout!* Super-Activity Book
The SWORD Adventure Book

* Available in Spanish

World Offices of
Kenneth Copeland Ministries

For more information about KCM and a free
catalog, please write the office nearest you:

Kenneth Copeland Ministries
Fort Worth, Texas 76192-0001

Kenneth Copeland Ministries
Locked Bag 2600
Mansfield Delivery Centre
QUEENSLAND 4122
AUSTRALIA

Kenneth Copeland Ministries
Post Office Box 15
BATH
BA1 1GD
ENGLAND

Kenneth Copeland Ministries
Private Bag X 909
FONTAINEBLEAU
2032
REPUBLIC OF
    SOUTH AFRICA

Kenneth Copeland Ministries
Post Office Box 378
Surrey
BRITISH COLUMBIA
V3T 5B6
CANADA

UKRAINE
L'VIV 290000
Post Office Box 84
Kenneth Copeland Ministries
L'VIV 290000
UKRAINE

We're Here for You!

Join Kenneth and Gloria Copeland, and the *Believer's Voice of Victory* broadcast, Monday through Friday and on Sunday each week, and learn how faith in God's Word can take your life from ordinary to extraordinary.

It's some of the most in-depth teaching you'll ever hear on subjects like faith and healing, deliverance and prosperity, protection and hope. And it's all designed to get you where you want to be—*on top!* The teachings are by some of today's best-known ministers, including Kenneth and Gloria Copeland, Jerry Savelle, Charles Capps, Creflo A. Dollar Jr., Kellie Copeland and Edwin Louis Cole.

So, whether it's before breakfast, during lunch or after a long day at the office, plan to make *Believer's Voice of Victory* a daily part of your life. And see for yourself how one word from God can change your life forever.

You can catch the *Believer's Voice of Victory* broadcast on the following cable and satellite channels:

Sunday
9-9:30 p.m. ET
Cable*/G5,
Channel 3—TBN

Monday through Friday
7-7:30 p.m. ET
Cable*/G1,
Channel 17—INSP

Monday through Friday
6-6:30 a.m. ET
Cable*/G5,
Channel 7—WGN

Monday through Friday
11-11:30 a.m. ET
Cable*/G5,
Channel 3—TBN

Monday through Friday
6:30-7 a.m. ET
Cable*/G5,
Channel 20—BET

Monday through Friday
6:30-7 a.m. ET
Cable*/W1,
Channel 7—Cornerstone TV

*Check your local listing for more times and stations in your area.

Believer's Voice of Victory

Nowhere else will you get a monthly dose of the inspired teaching and encouragement of Kenneth and Gloria Copeland than in the issues of the *Believer's Voice of Victory* magazine. Also included are real-life testimonies of God's miraculous power and divine intervention into the lives of people just like you! Featured guest ministers offer their latest revelation and godly instruction to encourage your faith.

If you would like to receive a FREE subscription to *Believer's Voice of Victory,* just send your name and address to:

Kenneth Copeland Ministries
Fort Worth, Texas 76192-0001
It's more than just a magazine—it's a ministry.

Shout!

...The faith-filled magazine just for kids!

Shout! The Voice of Victory for Kids is a Word-charged, action-packed, bimonthly magazine that's available FREE to kids everywhere!

Featuring *Wichita Slim* and *Commander Kellie and the Superkids*sm, *Shout!* is filled with colorful adventure comics, challenging games and puzzles, exciting short stories, solve-it-yourself mysteries and much more!!

So if you or some of your friends would like to receive a FREE subscription to *Shout!*, just send each kid's name, date of birth and complete address to:

Kenneth Copeland Ministries
Fort Worth, Texas 76192-0001

Or call:

1-800-359-0075
(9 a.m.-5 p.m. CT)

Stand up, sign up and get ready to *Shout!*

About the Authors

Kenneth and Gloria Copeland are best-selling authors of more than 60 books, such as the popular *Walk With God, Managing God's Mutual Funds* and *God's Will for You.* Together they have co-authored numerous books, including *Family Promises.* As founders of Kenneth Copeland Ministries in Fort Worth, Tex., Kenneth and Gloria are in their 31st year of circling the globe with the uncompromised Word of God, preaching and teaching a lifestyle of victory for every Christian.

Their daily *Believer's Voice of Victory* television broadcast now airs on more than 500 stations around the world. Their *Believer's Voice of Victory* and *Shout!* magazines are distributed to more than 1 million adults and children worldwide. Their international prison ministry reaches an average of 60,000 new inmates every year and receives more than 17,000 pieces of correspondence every month. Ken and Gloria Copeland have offices and staff in the United States, Canada, England, Australia, South Africa and the Ukraine. The Copelands' teaching materials found on the World Wide Web include stories on such topics as Marriage, the Holy Spirit, Money Management and Health and Healing. Their books, magazines, audiotapes and videotapes have been translated into more than 20 languages to reach the world with the God kind of love.

Learn more about Kenneth Copeland Ministries by visiting our website at:

www.kcm.org

The Harrison House Vision

Proclaiming the truth and the power
Of the Gospel of Jesus Christ
With excellence;
Challenging Christians to
Live victoriously,
Grow spiritually,
Know God intimately.